QUICK AND FIT: A BUSY PERSON'S DIET GUIDE AND WEIGHT LOSS ROADMAP

A Simple, Super Easy Diet Plan for Attaining Your Ideal Weight with 100+ Weight Loss Diet Recipes

Sarah Jordan, LD, CCN

COPYRIGHT PAGE

Copyright © 2023 by Sarah Jordan, LD, CCN

The information and recipes in Quick And Fit: A Busy Person's Diet Guide and Weight Loss Roadmap are not meant to replace professional medical or nutritional advice and are provided solely for educational reasons. The author and publisher disclaim all liability for any harm that may come from following the advice in this book. Before making any modifications to one's diet or beginning a program to lose weight, it is recommended that the reader seek the advice of a healthcare provider or nutritionist.

Table of Contents

CHAPTER I: WEIGHT LOSS FOR BUSY PEOPLE

In today's fast-paced world, weight reduction for business people is an important subject. It's not easy to put your health and weight reduction first when you have a demanding job, but doing so is essential to your long-term success and peak performance.

As a business professional, you should know the basics of weight reduction before you start your path. Calorie balance refers to the idea that one should expend an equal number of calories in their daily activities and through physical exercise as they take in through their diet. In order to lose weight, it is essential to generate a calorie deficit by cutting food consumption or increasing physical activity.

It's crucial to take an optimistic outlook and work toward attainable goals. Realize that losing weight and keeping it off requires time and work. Maintaining motivation and avoiding discouragement can be aided by setting attainable objectives and concentrating on the process rather than the final product. Long-term success requires developing a mentality of self-compassion and accepting failures as chances for growth.

Successful weight reduction for busy professionals requires time management methods. It's crucial to figure out how to fit healthy routines and time management into a hectic schedule. Planning and prepping healthy meals and snacks in advance might help you make better eating choices when you're pressed for time. Making healthy meal choices on the fly, such as when eating out or on business trips, might aid in weight reduction efforts.

Regular exercise and other forms of physical activity are crucial for health and weight reduction. Short exercises on the calendar or active breaks sprinkled throughout the day are just two examples of how to integrate exercise into a hectic schedule and still reap the benefits. Selecting fun and doable activities is essential when time is limited.

Successful weight reduction for business people requires addressing stress and emotional eating. Poor food selection and emotional eating, both of which are exacerbated by stress, can make it difficult to lose weight. Stress may be mitigated and improved coping mechanisms developed via the use of stress management strategies including mindfulness, meditation, and the pursuit of interests.

Sleep and recuperation should be prioritized for weight reduction, however this is rarely done. A good night's sleep is crucial to maintaining healthy hormone levels and general health. Establishing a regular bedtime routine, learning and using relaxation strategies, and providing a soothing atmosphere are all crucial elements.

The achievement of weight loss goals is significantly aided by accountability and support networks. For inspiration, accountability, and moral support on your quest to a healthier weight, consider enlisting the help of loved ones or coworkers. It might also be helpful to engage with a professional, such as a qualified nutritionist or personal trainer, or to join a support group that is dedicated to weight loss.

Losing weight involves more than just avoiding food. It's normal to hit a weight reduction plateau every once in a while. Here is a chance to take stock, make necessary course corrections, and maintain focus on the big picture.

If you want to keep the weight off and improve your health, you need to make adjustments to your eating and exercise habits that will last. The "yo-yo" diet cycle should be avoided at all costs in favor of long-term, sustainable lifestyle changes. Key components of retaining motivation and avoiding burnout include celebrating successes and engaging in self-care.

Successful weight loss for business professionals calls for a multifaceted strategy that incorporates knowledge of weight loss principles, goal setting, time management, food selection, exercise, stress management, sleep prioritization, seeking support, overcoming obstacles, and long-term maintenance of lifestyle changes. Business workers may lose weight, keep their careers going strong, and improve their health if they put health first and use these techniques.

Prioritizing health and weight loss amidst a busy professional lifestyle

A professional's hectic schedule might make it easier to put off caring for one's health and achieving weight reduction objectives. However, in order to sustain long-term success and general well-being, it is crucial to acknowledge the necessity of prioritizing health.

Taking care of one's health has far-reaching effects on one's mental and emotional wellness, in addition to the obvious physical benefits. Putting your health and weight reduction first may give you more drive, help you concentrate better, and boost your output at work. When we're healthy, our minds and bodies are in better sync, and that leads to more productivity and happiness on the job.

In addition, making health and weight reduction a top priority can aid in the avoidance of chronic diseases and the mitigation of associated risks. Heart disease, diabetes, and certain cancers are among the many health problems that may be avoided by exercising regularly and eating healthily. By making a commitment to our health today, we are taking preventative measures to ensure our happiness in the future.

Taking care of oneself is not egotistical. When we put our own wellness first, we inspire our friends, family, and coworkers to do the same. When we take care of ourselves, we are in a better position to help people in our life, both professionally and personally.

It may be necessary to make conscious decisions and develop techniques to incorporate good habits into a hectic schedule in order to achieve a healthy work-life balance. Practical methods of stress management, time management, healthy eating, and regular exercise are all examples. Consistently taking baby measures toward better health and weight loss might lead to big changes over time.

Putting health and weight reduction first, even in the middle of a hectic work life, is an investment in our future happiness and success. If we give our health the attention it deserves, we will be able to strike a balance between our work and personal life that will allow us to flourish.

Understanding Weight Loss Principles

Anyone who wants to lose weight and improve their health should first learn the fundamentals of weight loss. Calorie balance is the fundamental notion underlying successful weight loss. In other words, weight loss requires an energy deficit, wherein the number of calories taken in through food and drink is less than the number of calories burned off by exercise and normal metabolic processes. Because of the resulting calorie shortfall, the body will start using fat reserves as a source of fuel.

But cutting back on calories isn't the only key to losing weight. The quantity of calories ingested is not as important as their quality. A diet rich in whole foods, fruits, vegetables, lean meats, and healthy fats will help you feel full longer and improve your health in general.

Exercising regularly is also essential for successful weight loss. Consistent exercise and an increase in activity levels throughout the day have several metabolic benefits. To maximize weight reduction and enhance body composition, it is best to combine cardio for calorie burning with strength training.

In addition, dropping pounds is not a straight line. The rate at which a person loses weight depends on a number of factors, including genetics, metabolism, and body composition. Setting achievable objectives and welcoming the journey as a lifelong dedication to health and wellness is essential.

Quick cures and fad diets don't work, but a balanced and thoughtful approach to food and exercise does, leading to long-term weight reduction success. Changing to a healthier way of life demands doing it in baby steps. The secret is to ignore perfectionism and concentrate on making progress.

Learning the fundamentals of weight reduction enables people to make educated decisions and establish reasonable objectives. Individuals may lose weight and enhance their health, self-esteem, and quality of life by using a comprehensive strategy that includes calorie balance, healthy food, regular physical exercise, and an attitude of long-term commitment.

When attempting to lose weight, it is essential to create reasonable objectives and alter one's outlook. Realistically expecting rapid results is unrealistic, therefore it's important to keep this process in perspective. A lack of motivation and probable setbacks might result from setting objectives that are too lofty or impossible to achieve.

Instead, defining attainable goals increases the likelihood of long-term success. Realizing that, while outcomes may vary from person to person, a healthy rate of weight reduction is between one and two pounds per week is a good place to start. Individuals are more likely to stay motivated and keep moving forward toward their objectives if they divide them into smaller, more manageable chunks.

The ups and downs of weight reduction need not only reasonable expectations but also a mental shift. Keeping a hopeful and charitable frame of mind is essential. When people embrace themselves and show themselves compassion throughout the process, they may shift their attention from the number on the scale to their overall health and happiness.

Realizing that you've hit a brief snag or plateau is crucial. Missteps need not be viewed as setbacks, but rather as stepping stones to success. Building toughness and sticking with a task through tough times are two qualities that will serve you well.

The emphasis must also be shifted from "dieting" to a lifestyle that prioritizes health and wellness. A healthy connection with food and the body may be fostered by putting an emphasis on wholesome routines rather than extreme or temporary actions.

Consistency and toughness are also influenced by one's mindset. By viewing weight reduction as an opportunity for self-improvement, one may learn to be happy with even little victories, regardless of the number on the scale. The good effects of adopting a healthier lifestyle are reinforced when people celebrate successes that can't be measured on a scale, such as having more energy, being in better shape, or feeling more confident in themselves.

The keys to a successful weight reduction journey are a change in perspective and the establishment of reasonable objectives. Individuals may overcome obstacles, enjoy success in spite of setbacks, and keep making strides toward a better and happier life by adopting a mindset of self-compassion, building resilience, and centering their efforts on the long haul.

Time Management Strategies

If you want to lose weight or just start living healthier, you need to learn how to prioritize your time effectively. Individuals may prioritize their health and well-being despite the pressures of work and other obligations by careful time management.

Setting priorities and making a timetable is crucial. To do this, one must determine which activities are crucial and then set aside time for them. Schedules that include time for things like working out, making meals, and taking care of oneself help people give these priorities the care they need. Schedule them as though they were very necessary to avoid missing them or putting them off.

Maximizing productivity by taking on many tasks at once is another viable option. It is possible to save time by incorporating healthful practices into already planned tasks. Making the most of downtime by listening to instructional podcasts or audiobooks while running or cleaning is one example. Similarly, batch meal **Preparation** or the use of meal delivery services can facilitate healthy eating during the week without requiring additional time out of your busy schedule.

Another important part of efficient time management is getting rid of things that waste time. Realizing how much time you spend on screens (especially social media and television) and taking steps to reduce that time might free you up for other fulfilling activities. A more healthy equilibrium between work and play may be achieved by the deliberate establishment of limits and selection of activities during free time.

It's also important to maximize the time you have available at little intervals throughout the day. Short bouts of exercise, such as a quick stroll or desk exercises, can build up and contribute to overall fitness during breaks and lunch hours. It's also possible to improve one's state of mind and save time by doing so during one's commute by engaging in activities like practicing mindfulness, listening to informative podcasts, or engaging in deep breathing exercises.

Finally, it's important to ask for help and delegate duties. Time and tension may be saved by realizing it's okay to ask for help rather than trying to handle everything alone. Whether it's by sharing duties at home, getting the whole family involved in food prep, or reaching out to trusted friends and coworkers, having a strong support system is essential for efficient time management.

Effective time management techniques are crucial for achieving one's weight reduction and healthy lifestyle objectives despite a packed agenda. Individuals may maximize their time and establish a balanced lifestyle that promotes their well-being and weight loss journey by setting priorities and creating schedules, multitasking when feasible, avoiding time-wasting activities, making advantage of tiny pockets of time, and seeking help.

Effective techniques to optimize time and incorporate healthy habits into a busy schedule

Successful time management is essential for fitting in healthy routines while maintaining a full workload. Methods to save time and focus on health are provided below.

Planning and prioritizing can be used as a method. Make a concerted effort by scheduling in time for healthy routines and establishing concrete goals. Making a plan ensures that important activities, such as working exercise, meal planning on the weekends, and self-care, get the time and attention they require.

Utilizing little intervals of time throughout the day is another useful strategy. Use the time you have effectively rather than waiting for enormous blocks of free time. Some examples of this include using your travel time to practice mindfulness or yoga while stretching during a conference call.

Time can also be saved by simplifying repeated tasks. Choosing healthy, quick-to-prepare meals and making use of time-saving kitchen appliances or meal delivery services may make meal planning a breeze. High-intensity interval training (HIIT) and circuit training are two effective methods for maximizing calorie expenditure during exercise.

Delegating or outsourcing work might also help you save time. Think about getting a virtual assistant to help with paperwork, delegating certain duties to family members, or using a meal planning service. More time and effort may be put toward prioritizing health and well-being if tasks are split up.

Setting limits is another component of efficient time management. Master the art of politely declining invitations and declining unnecessary obligations. In order to make room for self-care and good behaviors, it may be essential to reduce time spent on other, less important chores.

Third, making better use of time may be facilitated by adopting technology. Take advantage of the convenient and effective training possibilities provided by fitness apps and internet platforms. Check out these healthy meal planning apps or websites for inspiration on fast and easy meals. Take advantage of your commute or downtime by listening to an audiobook or podcast to further your education.

Using these methods of time management, people may streamline their calendars and find time for physical activity despite their hectic lifestyles. Conscious decision making, prioritization, and time-saving strategies for improving well-being are the keys. Striking a balance between a rigorous schedule and a healthy lifestyle is attainable with careful **Preparation** and dedication.

Meal Planning and Preparation

Planning and preparing meals in advance are helpful ways to fit healthy eating into a hectic schedule. Planning and preparing meals ahead of time can help people save time, pick healthier options, and stick to their diets more consistently.

Making a weekly or monthly menu with a range of healthy and well-balanced meals is the first step in meal planning. Planning meals requires thinking about time and money constraints, as well as personal tastes and nutritional requirements. Individuals may save time and money by preparing meals in advance, since they will already have all the materials on hand.

The **Preparation** of meals follows the planning phase. Batch cooking, chopping vegetables, and pre-portioning **Ingredients** all take time that may be better spent elsewhere. Aside from freeing up time during the week, meal prepping also makes it less likely that you'll reach for quick and unhealthy fast food.

One easy way to save time in the kitchen is to prepare big quantities of pantry staples like healthy grains, meats, and roasted veggies. These may be made ahead of time, put in the fridge or freezer, and used as **Ingredients** for meals all week long. Also, you may save time and effort by preparing fruits, veggies, and nutritious snacks in individual serving containers.

Having a well-stocked pantry and fridge is an additional part of meal planning and preparation. It's far simpler to whip up quick and healthy meals if you keep pantry essentials like whole grains, lean meats, fruits, veggies, and healthy fats on hand.

Preparing meals ahead of time also helps with portion management. Individuals can better control their calorie intake and prevent overeating if they pre-portion their meals and snacks. Controlling one's portion sizes is essential for successful weight management and good health.

In addition, doing so allows you to try out different flavors and **Ingredients** as you plan and prepare meals. It empowers people to make more considered decisions about what they eat and how they prepare their meals.

Meal planning and **Preparation** may take some effort at first, but it pays off in the long run. Preparing nutritious meals ahead of time helps people save time, feel less pressure around mealtime, and maintain their health and weight reduction efforts. It helps people develop a more positive attitude about food, promotes mindful eating, and improves their odds of successfully sticking to a healthy eating plan despite time constraints.

Practical tips for planning and preparing nutritious meals ahead of time to avoid unhealthy food choices

Preparing healthy meals in advance is a great way to keep from making poor food decisions and promote a balanced diet. If you're not sure where to begin, consider these suggestions:

To get started, set aside some time once a week just for meal preparation. The weekend or any convenient time is fine for this. Take this opportunity to plan your weekly meals, make a shopping list, and peruse recipe sites.

Choose dishes that incorporate a wide variety of fruits, vegetables, whole grains, and lean meats to achieve a healthy balance of macronutrients (carbohydrates, proteins, and fats). The key to fulfilling and enjoyable meals is diversity.

After deciding what you'll eat for the week, write down what you'll need to buy at the grocery store. If you make a list before going grocery shopping, you're less likely to buy unhealthy snacks on the spur of the moment.

Plan to do your meal prep at a certain time every day. This may be done in a single weekend afternoon or a weeknight after work. Prepare your fruits and veggies for the week by cleaning, chopping, and plating them now. Precooked chicken, turkey, or tofu, as well as healthful grains like quinoa or brown rice, are more options.

Prepare your meals in advance by purchasing meal-prep containers. Separate the finished meats, grains, and veggies into separate containers. If you're ever in a pinch for time and need to grab something quickly, this is a great alternative.

You may save time and money by cooking in bulk or producing extra of each meal. This manner, you may eat healthfully without having to do any more cooking beyond reheating.

Utilize the gadgets in your kitchen that will save you time while cooking. Appliances like the slow cooker and the instant pot simplify and speed up the cooking process.

Preparing healthy meals ahead of time increases the likelihood that you will eat them and decreases the likelihood that you would choose less healthy options because they are more inconvenient. Additionally, it helps you remain on track with your diet even on hectic days by removing the burden of picking what to eat.

Smart Food Choices on the Go

If you want to keep up a healthy diet and make progress toward your weight reduction goals despite your hectic schedule, you need to learn how to make good meal choices on the go. Here are some tips to keep in mind when making healthy food choices away from home:

- Take a few moments before leaving the house to arrange your day's meals and snacks. Think about when you'll need to eat while on the road due to your schedule. If you're planning ahead, you'll be less likely to resort to unhealthy fast food or vending machine snacks.

- Snacks on the Go: Make healthy, on-the-go snacks ahead of time and pack them. To keep you going strong all day long, bring some healthy snacks like these: fresh fruit, chopped veggies, almonds, seeds, or granola bars you made yourself. You won't be hungry for long since these snacks are packed with energy, fiber, and minerals.

- Select Meals and Snacks High in Protein

  Protein is an essential food that aids in promoting satiety and maintaining stable blood sugar levels. For protein, try pre-packaged portions of lean meats, Greek yogurt, string cheese, and hard-boiled eggs. You may eat them as side dishes or as a snack on their own.

- Choose whole foods over processed or packaged ones as much as possible. Fresh fruits and vegetables, whole grains, and lean meats all provide a wide variety of essential nutrients while also being relatively low in harmful fats, salt, and sugar.

- Make use of the salad bars and deli areas that can be found in many supermarkets, cafés, and restaurants. Benefit from these alternatives and create a well-rounded meal by using different veggies, lean meats, and nutritious grains. Dressings and toppings may quickly rack up the calories, so pick healthier options or ask for them on the side.

- Maintaining an adequate water intake is crucial to good health and can serve as a useful tool in controlling hunger and avoiding binge eating. Get yourself a refillable water bottle and sip from it frequently during the day. Herbal teas without added sugar are a great choice, as is infusing water with fresh fruits and herbs.

- Take the time to study the labels and nutritional information before buying any prepackaged snacks or on-the-go meals. Try to find foods that are low in harmful additives like sugar, salt, and fat. Look for items that are rich in healthy nutrients including fiber, protein, and healthy fats.

Choosing nutritious meals when on the road requires striking a balance between time and effort. You can still provide your body with the nourishment it needs even when you're on the go and pressed for time by planning ahead, carrying healthy snacks, selecting whole foods, and being attentive of nutritional value.

Guidance on making healthy food choices when eating out, ordering takeout, or traveling for work

Eating well when dining out, ordering takeout, or traveling for work can be difficult, but with little planning, it is easy to maintain a balanced diet despite these obstacles. Some advice on how to improve your diet:

Study and prepare ahead of time: It's a good idea to check out the menu online before going out to eat or placing a takeout order. You may now plan your meal in advance thanks to the availability of online menus at many eateries. Try to eat more lean meats, veggies, and healthy grains. You may make a smarter choice and steer clear of less healthy impulse buys by preparing ahead.

Pick Wisely: When dining out, go for grilled, steamed, roasted, or baked dishes rather than fried or breaded ones. Salads, stir-fries, and grilled fish and chicken are great examples of vegetable- and lean-protein-rich recipes that you should prioritize. Never be afraid to make a better choice, such as ordering a side salad instead of french fries or switching to whole grain bread instead of white bread.

Restaurants typically provide more food than is necessary; this must be stopped. You might ask for a half serving or split a meal with a coworker. You might also request a takeout container at the start of your dinner and divide up portions to take home for later. You can keep your weight in check and prevent yourself from overeating if you only watch your portions.

Sauces and dressings are often used to enhance the flavor of a food, but they may add a lot of extra calories, harmful fats, and sugars if you're not careful. You may better regulate the calories and fat you consume by asking for sauces, dressings, and condiments on the side. To add taste without adding extra calories, try vinaigrettes, salsas, or lemon juice.

Choose Your Sides and Drinks Wisely Consider the accompaniments and drinks carefully. Substitute steamed veggies, a side salad, or a baked potato for fried choices like fries or onion rings. Avoid empty-calorie drinks like sugary sodas and alcoholic beverages in favor of healthier options like water, unsweetened tea, or sparkling water.

Bring Your Own Snacks: Instead of buying junk food from a vending machine or a convenience store when you're on the road for business or pleasure, bring some nutritious snacks with you. Grab some fresh produce, some cut-up veggies, some almonds, or some homemade granola bars. These snacks are perfect for filling you up in between meals and keeping you from making unhealthy, hasty decisions.

It's always about making the most advantageous decisions you can. Eating healthily whether dining out, ordering takeaway, or traveling for work just requires some forethought, a focus on whole foods, and the management of portion sizes.

CHAPTER III: EXERCISE AND PHYSICAL ACTIVITY

Regular exercise and other forms of physical activity are essential to everyone's well-being. There are various physiological and psychological advantages to maintaining an exercise routine.

Exercising helps with weight control and also aids in keeping a healthy body composition. Weight reduction and maintenance can benefit from its ability to boost metabolism, burn calories, and promote lean muscle growth.

Having a healthy heart and good blood flow is only one of the many benefits of a regular workout routine. It's been shown to decrease blood pressure, increase good cholesterol, and minimize the likelihood of developing heart disease. Cardiovascular health can be greatly improved by regular vigorous exercise such brisk walking, running, cycling, or swimming.

In addition, regular exercise is an important tool for stress reduction and overall mental health and wellness. Endorphins, or "feel-good" chemicals, are released in response to physical exercise, elevating mood and decreasing anxious or depressed sensations. It's a healthy alternative for dealing with stress and increasing mental toughness.

Bone health may be preserved and bone loss associated with aging can be avoided with regular exercise. Bone density is increased and the risk of osteoporosis is decreased by weight-bearing workouts including walking, jogging, and strength training.

Exercise has many positive effects on the body, but it also helps the mind and the brain. In elderly people, it has been associated to better memory, sharper attention, and slower mental deterioration.

Finding things that you love and can realistically include into your routine is crucial when trying to fit fitness into a hectic schedule. Shorter, more intense exercises, spreading out physical activity throughout the day, and finding novel ways to incorporate movement into routine chores, like using the stairs instead of the elevator or parking further away, are all viable options.

Never forget that some physical activity is always preferable to none at all. Begin with manageable objectives, then build up your workout duration and intensity over time. Exercise on a consistent basis; this might be three times per week or every day, depending on your schedule and current fitness level.

Finally, physical activity and exercise have many positive effects on health and well-being. Maintaining a regular exercise regimen has several long-term health benefits, including but not limited to weight control, cardiovascular health, stress reduction, and enhanced cognitive performance. If you want to reap the benefits of an active lifestyle, you need to choose things that you like and make them a priority.

Strategies to incorporate exercise into a busy routine, including short workouts, desk exercises, and active breaks

Although it may appear difficult to fit exercise into a hectic schedule, it is feasible to do so with some forward thinking and innovative solutions. In order to include exercise into your hectic schedule, consider the following options:

Focus on shorter, more intensive workouts as opposed to long, leisurely sessions. Workouts like high-intensity interval training (HIIT) can improve cardiovascular fitness and muscle strength in as little as 15 to 20 minutes. Try to find exercises that train many muscle groups at once so that you may get the most out of your workout time and burn the most calories.

Take advantage of little breaks during the day to perform some desk exercises. Stretching, sitting leg lifts, and shoulder rolls are all great ways to release tension in the body, increase blood flow, and perk up your energy levels. When sitting for extended durations, set reminders or utilize smartphone applications to remind you to get up and move about every so often.

Don't just sit about or look at your phone during your breaks; get up and move around a bit. Get some exercise by going for a brisk stroll around the workplace, using the stairs, or doing a bodyweight circuit in the park. These exercises not only improve your body, but also your mind and spirit, allowing you to return to work invigorated and ready to get more done.

Attempt to find ways to include physical activity into your already busy schedule. In the case of a conference call or online meeting, for instance, you might pace the room or perform basic exercises like squats and lunges without disrupting the flow of the conversation. If you want to work out your muscles while at your computer, you may use a stability ball or a standing desk.

Consistency is the most important, even if lengthier workouts are difficult to fit into a hectic schedule. Maintain a consistent exercise schedule, even if it consists of shorter sessions. Shorter workouts spread out throughout the week are preferable than lengthier workouts that are less frequent. Workouts should ideally be done before work or at lunch to minimize interference from other obligations.

Make the most of your weekends by sleeping in later or engaging in more strenuous physical activity. Take use of the time by going on a stroll, riding your bike, or attending a fitness class. To spend quality time with loved ones and get some exercise, organize a fun group activity.

Keep in mind that any physical activity is better than none. Don't discount the value of squeezing in a few minutes of exercise here and there; little things add up. Successfully incorporating exercise into your hectic schedule and reaping the physical and emotional health advantages of regular physical activity requires being purposeful and finding inventive methods to stay active.

Stress Management and Emotional Eating

Emotional eating and stress management go hand in hand, therefore it's important to recognize the connection between the two. Many people use food as a means of emotional regulation and solace when they are under stress. The detrimental repercussions on one's mental and physical health from this pattern of eating are well-documented.

Effective stress management and the elimination of emotional eating need the cultivation of coping strategies that do not involve food. Reducing stress and the desire to use food as consolation can be accomplished by the practice of activities like exercise, meditation, or deep breathing. These actions are excellent for lowering stress levels and increasing relaxation. Stress may be reduced and negative feelings can be channeled constructively via regular exercise, social interaction, and other forms of self-care.

Stress and emotional eating can be difficult to control without the help of loved ones or a therapist. Finding healthy methods to deal with stress can be greatly aided by talking to someone who understands and can provide support. Additional ideas and approaches to properly handle these difficulties might be obtained from therapists or counselors that specialize in stress management and emotional eating.

Emotional eating is a vicious cycle, but practicing mindful eating can help stop it. It means paying attention to the feelings and sensations you experience when you consume. A better connection with food may be fostered by learning to recognize the signals of hunger and fullness, chewing food thoroughly, and eating mindfully. Individuals can learn to distinguish between physical hunger and emotional desires by paying attention to the experience of eating and tuning into the body's signals.

Individuals can interrupt the pattern of emotional eating by actively managing stress and finding healthy methods to cope with emotions. Keep in mind that your path will be different from anybody else's, and that the goal is to identify the methods that work best for you. It is possible to manage stress, address emotional eating, and develop a healthy relationship with food with time, compassion, and the help of loved ones or trained specialists.

Techniques for managing stress and overcoming emotional eating triggers in a professional setting

In a professional situation, it might be difficult but not impossible to manage stress and overcome emotional eating triggers. Here are some strategies that might help you deal with challenging circumstances:

Take care of yourself first. Relax with some deep breathing exercises or some light stretching at regular intervals during the day. Go for a stroll or do any other form of physical exercise that helps you relax and get some much-needed time to yourself during your lunch break.

Methods of dealing with stress, such as setting priorities and managing time, should be put into practice. Create smaller, more achievable projects, establish reasonable deadlines, and delegate if you can. Reducing stress and avoiding the buildup of pressure that can lead to emotional eating can be accomplished via prudent time management.

Find alternative, non-food ways to deal with stress. Use activities such as writing, chatting to a close friend or colleague, or indulging in a creative pastime to relieve tension and express feelings.

These actions can help you feel better and work through your feelings without resorting to food.

Even if you're at work, try to eat with more awareness. Mind your hunger and fullness cues, eat gently, and enjoy every meal. Choose healthful foods and consume them with purpose rather than mindlessly munching at your desk.

Make sure your office is a positive place to work. Discuss your stress management and emotional eating objectives and struggles with your coworkers or boss. Wellness programs and stress-reduction events, including yoga and mindfulness classes, may do wonders for a company's morale and productivity.

Get help from experts if you feel you need it. Consider seeing a counselor or therapist who specializes in stress management or disordered eating if stress and emotional eating continue despite your best efforts. They'll be able to customize their advice and methods to your unique situation.

Keep in mind that it takes time and self-compassion to learn to deal with stress and overcome the triggers that lead to emotional eating. Discover what works for you and modify your approach to suit your specific working environment; everyone's path is different. Using these methods, you may improve your ability to handle stress, create more harmony in your personal life, and achieve more success in your career.

Getting enough rest is essential to your health and well-being. Restorative sleep is necessary for your body, mind, and spirit. It helps the body mend torn tissues, recall previously learned information, balance hormones, and fortify the immune system.

Establishing a regular sleep schedule is beneficial for both sleep quality and recovery. Establish a routine by maintaining a consistent time for going to bed and waking up, especially on the weekends. Make use of activities like reading, having a warm bath, or practicing relaxation techniques like deep breathing or meditation as part of your nightly routine to assist your body know it's time to wind down and get some shut-eye.

It's also important to make your space conducive to sleeping. Maintain a calm, dark, and peaceful atmosphere in your bedroom. Get yourself a supportive mattress and pillows to ensure a restful night's sleep. You should limit your use of electronic devices before bedtime since the blue light they generate might mess with your body's internal clock. White noise machines, earplugs, and blackout curtains can all help drown out distracting sounds from the outside world.

Putting sleep hygiene first is crucial for getting a good night's sleep. Caffeine and nicotine are stimulants that should be avoided in the hours before night. Reduce your alcohol intake because it might cause sleep disruptions. Maintain a regular exercise routine, but stop exercising several hours before night to give your body time to relax.

Learn to value other means of rejuvenation in addition to sleep. Take frequent breaks from your day-to-day activities, and especially from any mental or physical labor that you may be performing. Including mindfulness practice, hobbies, and time in nature into your routine can help you unwind and recharge. Find things to do that make you happy and help you relax; doing so will aid in your health and speed your recovery.

Keep in mind the critical role that rest and rejuvenation play in maintaining good health. You may improve your physical and mental performance, your sense of well-being, and your ability to deal with the challenges of everyday life by making sleep a priority, creating a regular sleep regimen, and using recovery procedures.

The importance of quality sleep and strategies to improve sleep patterns for better weight management

When it comes to maintaining a healthy weight, nothing is more crucial than getting a good night's sleep. Inadequate sleep has been associated with a higher probability of gaining weight and becoming obese. Better weight control may be greatly aided by recognizing the significance of sleep and adopting techniques to enhance sleep habits.

Important physiological functions, such as hormone modulation, cellular repair, and metabolic regulation, all take place when we sleep. The hormones ghrelin and leptin, which regulate feelings of fullness and hunger, can become unbalanced when we don't get enough quality sleep, leading to an increase in hunger and a desire for unhealthy, high-calorie, carbohydrate-rich foods. This might make it more challenging to avoid tempting but harmful foods and stick to a healthy eating plan.

Several methods can help with both sleep quality and weight control. A regular bedtime and morning routine should be established first. This includes weekends. This improves the quality of your sleep and helps your body's internal clock adjust.

It's critical to make sure you have a comfortable place to sleep. Make sure you have a quiet, dark, and warm bedroom to relax in. You should think about getting a good quality mattress and pillows that will help you get a good night's sleep. Reduce your use of electronic devices before bedtime since the blue light they generate can prevent melatonin from being produced. Instead, wind down with some quiet time before bed, whether that's reading, light stretching, or meditating.

Establishing a soothing habit before bed might help your body understand that it's time to shut down. Stay away from coffee and nicotine as close to bedtime as possible. Try some deep breathing exercises or a nice, warm bath to help you wind down and get some shut-eye instead.

Better sleep and a more manageable weight are two additional benefits of a regular workout routine. Try to get in some exercise during the day, but stop working out at least a couple hours before night. This helps your body prepare for sleep by easing into a state of relaxation.

Finally, reducing stress is crucial for maintaining a healthy weight and enhancing sleep quality. Disrupted sleep and poor dietary choices are two negative outcomes of stress. Adopt strategies for dealing with stress, such as deep breathing, meditation, or spending time with loved ones.

Better sleep and overall weight control efforts are aided by stress management strategies.

Improved weight control requires both awareness of the need of quality sleep and the implementation of interventions to enhance sleep patterns. Better sleep and better results in maintaining a healthy weight may be achieved by a combination of regular exercise, a relaxing bedtime ritual, a relaxing bedroom atmosphere, and stress management. Prioritizing sleep can help people achieve their health and fitness objectives, including losing weight.

Accountability and Support Systems

Successful weight management is just one area of life where accountability and support systems may make all the difference. Having others to hold you responsible and give motivation may be invaluable in helping you remain on track and accomplish your objectives.

Working with a coach, enrolling in a support group, or teaming up with a friend or family member who has similar objectives are all great ways to hold yourself accountable. Being answerable to another person instills in us a strong desire to see through our stated goals. As it helps to build a feeling of structure and dedication to healthy activities, this can be very helpful in weight management.

Having a group of people who can relate to your struggles and celebrate your triumphs on the road to weight loss is invaluable. They give a place to talk about problems, get help from others, and celebrate successes together. Practical solutions, accountability check-ins, and a sense of belonging and community are just a few examples of how support systems may increase motivation and resilience.

Self-accountability is just as crucial as having a strong external support system. In order to keep one's motivation and attention, it is helpful to create specific goals, keep track of one's progress, and constantly reflect on one's successes and failures. Tools like diet and exercise diaries, goal trackers, and smartphone applications with reminders and progress tracking can help people be more accountable to themselves.

The chance of success in maintaining a healthy weight can be considerably increased when internal and external responsibility and support networks are combined. By providing a feeling of structure, encouragement, and assistance along the way, these systems help people achieve and sustain success over the long haul.

Finding and using accountability and support structures that fit one's own unique situation and preferences is crucial. Finding the correct support system, whether through group meetings, a workout partner, or professional advice, may make a huge difference in the success of weight control attempts. Remember that everyone's path is different, and that having accountability and support networks in place may give you the push you need to get through tough times, maintain your motivation, and see your efforts through to the end.

Overcoming Plateaus and Challenges

Obstacles and plateaus are inevitable on the road to weight loss, but they may be surmounted with determination and planning. It's vital to keep in mind that growth plateaus are a natural part of any process, even if they can be frustrating and demoralizing when they occur. The following are some methods for getting through stagnation and overcoming obstacles:

Check your motivations and strategy first. Examine your present tactics to see whether any changes are required. You may do this by trying out new forms of exercise, adjusting your caloric intake, or switching up your current regimen. When you hit a stalemate in your development, don't be afraid to shake things up a bit.

Next, you should give some thought to keeping a more detailed diet and activity journal. Maintaining a food diary can help you keep track of what you eat and reveal hidden sources of excess calories. Mind your eating habits and focus on reducing portion sizes. You should also examine your fitness program to make sure you're pushing yourself hard enough and adding enough variation to avoid a rut.

Strength training is useful and should be implemented. Increasing your metabolic rate and aiding in weight reduction, strength exercise helps you gain lean muscle mass. Lifting weights or using resistance bands are two examples of resistance workouts that can help you build muscle and speed up your metabolism.

Keeping your stress levels in check is also crucial. Weight loss efforts might be hampered by the negative effects of stress on hormone regulation and appetite. Find effective methods of dealing with stress, such as meditation, yoga, or hobbies that allow you to unwind and relax.

Learn to ask for help and be accountable. Discuss your difficulties with a close confidant, member of your family, or a group of like-minded people. Based on their own experiences, they can provide words of encouragement, direction, and advise. Having someone you can trust on to keep you motivated and accountable during the rough times is essential.

Finally, have compassion and patience for yourself. Constantly encountering roadblocks and plateaus is par for the course. Focus on non-number triumphs, including higher energy and fitness levels, rather than the number on the scale to celebrate. Keep in mind that maintaining a healthy weight is a lifelong journey with minor bumps along the way. Trust the process and keep your sights set on your objectives.

You may overcome weight management obstacles by adjusting your strategy, keeping a progress journal, including strength exercise, dealing with stress, getting help, and showing yourself compassion. Always remember that you are getting closer to your objectives as you go forward in your efforts.

Maintaining Weight Loss and Sustainable Lifestyle Changes

Long-term success and health depend on the ability to keep off lost weight and stick with healthier habits in the long run. Achieving and maintaining a healthy weight involves more than just cutting back on calories and hitting the gym.

To keep the weight off for good, it's important to change your thinking from that of a diet to that of a lifetime change. To do this, you need alter your diet and exercise routine in a way that is sustainable over time. Dietary emphasis should be placed on a variety of entire, nutrient-dense foods, with room for variation and the odd indulgence. Avoid fad diets that are hard to maintain and might make you feel deprived.

Keeping up with a regular exercise routine is essential for good health and weight maintenance. Make time for the things that bring you joy every day. Consistency is key, so make it a priority to exercise your body on a daily basis, whether that means walking, running, cycling, dancing, or attending fitness classes. Alternating between different types of physical activity keeps you from becoming bored and improves your fitness by using different muscle groups.

Keeping a good frame of mind is also crucial. Practice self-compassion and acknowledge that progress is more important than perfection. Plan for success, not failure, and enjoy the small wins along the road. Keep in mind that failures are normal and expected along the way. Take use of these setbacks as learning experiences.

Keeping yourself around by positive people may have a dramatic effect on how far you get in life.

Make an effort to associate with people who share your values and will help you stay motivated and on track. Share your plight with your loved ones and ask them to help you out. Participate in communal health-enhancing pursuits like preparing and sharing healthy meals or going for walks.

Make sure your routines are consistent with your long-term objectives by evaluating them frequently. It's important to take stock of your eating habits, exercise schedule, and stress management strategies on a regular basis to make any required improvements. Maintain awareness of your eating habits, including the signals your body sends for hunger and fullness, and make deliberate decisions that benefit your health.

Finally, seek continuing help to keep you motivated and knowledgeable. Go to events like seminars and workshops, read books and articles, and talk to experts for advice and motivation. Join a community of people who understand what you're going through and have been through the same things you have. Having meaningful interactions with others may be a source of motivation, responsibility, and new perspectives.

Commitment, persistence, and a positive frame of mind are necessary for maintaining weight reduction and long-term lifestyle improvements. Adopt a middle ground, put your own needs first, and be kind with yourself. Achieving long-term weight control and reaping the rewards of a sustainable and meaningful lifestyle takes time, persistence, and the adoption of healthy behaviors.

Guidance on sustaining weight loss achievements, creating healthy habits, and making long-term lifestyle changes

Celebrating Success and Self-Care

Rejoicing in one's achievements and making self-care a top priority are crucial elements of a successful and long-lasting weight loss journey. Motivating yourself and reinforcing good habits may be as simple as acknowledging and enjoying even the smallest of victories.

Don't forget to stop and enjoy small victories along the path. Plan out your progress and celebrate with non-food indulgences like a day at the spa, new training clothes, or a day off to rest and rejuvenate rather than food. Marking and commemorating these achievements can serve as powerful reminders of the strides you've made toward your objectives.

Self-care is just as important as celebrating victories when it comes to sustaining mental and physical health. The mind, body, and spirit all benefit from self-care practices, which also serve to restore your vitality. Whether it's mindfulness meditation, a relaxing bubble bath, a good book, or quality time with loved ones, prioritizing these activities can help you relax and enjoy life more. Self-care activities not only help you relax, but they also help you have a good outlook and build resilience when life becomes tough.

Take care of your body; it's an important part of self-care. Getting enough sleep is crucial to your health and weight maintenance efforts. Establishing a regular nighttime routine and following it will help you get the peaceful slumber you need. Eat healthy, natural meals that will keep you energized and help your body function at its best. Drink plenty of water, keep moving, and pay attention to your body.

Self-compassion is also essential during the process of losing weight. Have compassion for yourself and see your flaws and failures as lessons. Instead of torturing yourself with negative thoughts, try encouraging yourself. Be as patient and nice to yourself as you would be to a loved one or close friend.

You may create a supportive and encouraging setting for long-term weight control by focusing on yourself and recognizing your achievements. These actions not only benefit your body, but also your state of mind and heart. To practice self-care is not egotistical; rather, it is an investment in your long-term well-being. As you go forward on the way to a better and more satisfying life, it's important to embrace the journey, celebrate your victories, and create a positive connection with yourself.

CHAPTER V: DIET PLAN AND RECIPES FOR SUPER EASY WEIGHT LOSS AS A BUSY PERSON

Rice Cooker Orange Upside-Down Cake

Ingredients

for 8 servings

- ¼ cup cream cheese (50 g), room temperature

- ½ cup sugar (100 g), plus 1 tablespoon, divided

- 2 large eggs

- 1 orange, washed

- 1 tablespoon lemon juice

- 1 cup pancake mix (150 g)

• ¼ cup butter (50 g), melted, plus more for greasing pan

Preparation

1. In a large bowl, combine the cream cheese and 100 g (½ cup) of the sugar. Add the eggs and whisk until combined.

2. Zest one half of the orange over the batter. Add the lemon juice and whisk to combine.

3. Add the pancake mix and melted butter, and whisk until the batter is smooth.

4. Brush the bowl of the rice cooker with melted butter.

5. Sprinkle the remaining tablespoon of sugar on the inside of the bowl so that it is well coated.

6. Slice the orange into 7 thin slices and lay on the inside of the bowl.

7. Pour the batter over the oranges, and cook for 40 minutes.

8. Remove the bowl of the rice cooker and place a plate over the top. Carefully flip the bowl upside-down so that the cake slides onto on the plate with the orange slices on top.

9. Enjoy!

Vegan Egg

Ingredients

for 12 eggs

Yolk

• 1 cup kabocha squash (125 g), steamed and mashed

• 3 tablespoons canola oil

• 12 tablespoons filtered water, cold, divided

• 1 teaspoon kala namak, Himalayan black salt

• ½ teaspoon kosher salt

• 1 tablespoon cornstarch

White

• 8 oz silken tofu (225 g), tofu

• 3 tablespoons rice flour

• 3 tablespoons filtered water, cold

• ½ teaspoon kala namak, Himalayan black salt

• 2 tablespoons full-fat coconut milk

Assembly

• 4 tablespoons canola oil, divided, for frying

• kosher salt, to taste

• black pepper, freshly ground, to taste

Preparation

1. Make the yolk: In a food processor or high-powered blender, combine the kabocha squash, canola oil, 10 tablespoons of water, the black salt, and kosher salt. Blend until completely smooth, about 1 minute, stopping to scrape down the sides as necessary. Transfer to a medium pot.

2. In a small bowl, whisk together the remaining 2 tablespoons of water and the cornstarch. Add to the yolk mixture.

3. Bring the yolk mixture to a low boil over medium-low heat, whisking constantly, until the mixture thickens to the consistency of pudding, 3-4 minutes.

4. Transfer the yolk mixture to a medium bowl and refrigerate until cooled completely, about 30 minutes.

5. While the yolk mixture cools, make the white: In a blender, combine the tofu, rice flour, water, black salt, coconut milk, and kosher salt. Blend until completely smooth. Transfer to a liquid measuring cup and set aside.

6. Using a ½ ounce domed silicone mold, divide the yolk mixture evenly between the cups. Refrigerate for 3 hours, until the yolks are set. (If you don't have a silicone mold, a tablespoon measure works well here).

7. Remove the yolks from the molds. Set on a paper towel-lined plate.

8. Heat 2 teaspoons of canola oil in a small skillet over medium heat. Pour about 1½-2 tablespoons of

the egg white mixture into the skillet. Spread around slightly to get an 'egg white' shape. Place a yolk, flat side down, on the white. Cover the skillet with a lid and reduce the heat to low. Cook for 3-4 minutes, until the edges of the white are very lightly browned and the yolk is warmed through. Repeat with remaining white and yolks, adding more oil to the pan as needed.

9. Season the "eggs" lightly with salt and pepper, then serve.

10. Enjoy!

Chewy Oatmeal Breakfast Bars To-go

Ingredients

for 8 servings

• 1 cup almond butter (240 g)

• ½ cup maple syrup (110 g)

• ½ cup almond milk (120 mL)

• 1 teaspoon vanilla

• 2 ½ cups rolled oats (250 g)

• 1 cup brown rice cereal (30 g)

• ½ cup slivered almond (35 g)

• ½ cup dried cranberry (65 g)

• ½ cup dark chocolate (85 g)

Drizzle

• ¼ cup dark chocolate (40 g), melted

Preparation

1. Preheat oven to 325°F (160°C).

2. Combine wet **Ingredients** together in a large bowl.

3. Then add in all the remaining dry ingredients.

4. Add mixture into a 8x8 inch (20x20 cm) baking pan lined with greased parchment paper. Firmly press down mixture until it is one smooth layer. (If you grease the spatula as well it will prevent the mixture from sticking to it!)

5. Bake 15-20 minutes, or until golden brown. Let cool 10 minutes.

6. Drizzle top with melted dark chocolate. Chill for 30 minutes, or until dark chocolate is solid.

7. Cut into 8 equal pieces.

8. Wrap each bar in parchment paper or foil.

9. Store in the freezer for up to 3 months or in the refrigerator up to 1 week.

10. Enjoy!

Easy Rice Cooker Green Tea Cake

Ingredients

for 6 servings

• 1.7 oz white chocolate (80 g)

• ¼ cup sugar (60 g)

• ¾ cup milk (200 mL)

• 2 eggs

• 2 cups flour (200 g)

• 3 ½ tablespoons matcha green tea powder

• 1 tablespoon baking powder

Garnish

• 1.7 oz white chocolate (50 g)

• strawberry

• blueberry

Preparation

1. Warm up milk until almost boiling.

2. In a bowl, put in the white chocolate and sugar, then pour over warm milk and mix until chocolate is melted.

3. Add 2 eggs and mix.

4. Add flour, green tea powder, and baking powder into the mixture. Pour into the rice cooker pan and cook for 1 hour.

5. Take the cake out from the pan and let it cool.

6. Glaze with melted white chocolate, then add the strawberries and blueberries.

7. Enjoy!

Sweet Sesame Dumplings (Tangyuan)

Ingredients

for 4 servings

Filling

• 1 cup black sesame seeds (150 g), toasted, ground

• ¼ cup powdered sugar (25 g)

• 1 ½ tablespoons unsalted butter

Dough

• 2 cups glutinous rice flour (250 g), plus more for dusting

• 1 cup warm water (240 mL)

For Cooking

• 2 tablespoons sugar

• 1 tablespoon osmanthus, dried flower

Preparation

1. Make the filling: In a medium bowl, combine the ground black sesame seeds, powdered sugar and melted butter. Mix until well combined. Roll 1 tablespoon scoops of the mixture into balls. Set aside.

2. Make the dough: Add the rice flour to a medium bowl. Gradually add the water and mix with your hands until the dough comes together.

3. On a lightly floured surface, turn out the dough. Shape into a ball and cut in half. Roll the dough into 2 logs, then cut into about 16 2-3-ounce (55G -85G) portions.

4. Flatten a dough portion in your palm and add a sesame ball to the center. Encase the filling with the dough and roll into a ball. Repeat with the remaining ingredients.

5. Bring a large pot of water to boil. Add the sugar and osmanthus flower. Drop the dumplings into the boiling water. Gently stir so they don't stick to the bottom of the pot. Cook until the dumplings float to the surface, then remove from the pot.

6. Serve the dumplings in a bowl with the cooking liquid.

7. Enjoy!

Jasmine's Snack Board

Ingredients

for 4 servings

Prawn Crackers

• 2 cups canola oil (480 mL), for frying

• 1 box prawn-flavored chips

Spam Musubi

• 2 tablespoons canola oil

- ½ can Spam®, halved lengthwise

- 2 tablespoons water

- 2 tablespoons soy sauce

- 2 tablespoons sugar, plus 2 teaspoons, divided

- ½ teaspoon kosher salt

- 2 tablespoons rice vinegar

- 1 ⅓ cups sushi rice (265 g), cooked

- 4 strips nori, 2 in (5 cm)

California Roll

- canola oil, for greasing

- 2 cups sushi rice (400 g), cooked, seasoned with 2 tablespoons of rice vinegar

- 8 pieces imitation crab

- 1 avocado, thinly sliced

- 1 small cucumber, cut into machsticks

- 4 sheets sushi-grade nori, 8½ x 7½

Assembly

- 1 package pan-fried dumplings, 24 ounce (700 G)

- 2 cups garlic edamame (320 g)

- 4 scallion pancakes, cut into triangles

- 1 large red dragon fruit, peeled and diced

- 4 pineapple cakes

- 4 probiotic yogurt drinks

- 8 pieces assorted mochi

- 1 loaf mujigae-tteok loaf, sliced

- 2 strawberry flavored Hello Panda cookies, 9 ounce (260 grams)

- 4 choco pies

- 1 cara cara orange, large, sliced

- 2 Mandarin orange slices

- 1 large asian pear, sliced

Preparation

1. Make the prawn crackers: Heat the oil in a large heavy-bottomed pan over medium heat until the temperature reaches 325°F (160°C). Line a plate with paper towels and set nearby.

2. Place 8–10 chips in a slotted spoon or spider. Gently lower them into the hot oil and stir gently. As the chips begin to float to the surface, quickly remove from the oil before they scorch or burn. Carefully shake off any excess oil, and then place on the lined plate. Continue frying the remaining chips.

3. Make the spam musubi: Heat the canola oil in a large nonstick skillet over medium-high heat. Add the Spam and cook for 2–3 minutes per side, until golden brown and crispy.

4. In a small bowl, whisk together the water, soy sauce, and 2 tablespoons of sugar.

5. Reduce the heat to low and pour the soy sauce mixture into the skillet. Cook until the sauce is bubbly and thick and coats the Spam evenly, turning as needed, about 5 minutes total. Remove the pan from the heat.

6. In a medium bowl, whisk together the remaining 2 teaspoons sugar, salt, and vinegar. Add the cooked sushi rice and stir to combine.

7. Lay a strip of nori, shiny side down, on a clean surface. Place the box of the musubi press on top. Add ⅓ cup of the seasoned rice to the box and press

down with the plunger. Lay a piece of Spam on top of the rice and press down firmly. Lift the box to release the Spam and rice. Wrap the nori around the stack, using a wet finger to seal the nori.

8. Make the California rolls: Lightly grease the inner chamber of a sushi bazooka with canola oil.

9. Add ½ cup of the seasoned sushi rice to each half of the inner chamber and use the plunger to create a divot down the length of each side of rice. Arrange half of the crab, avocado, and cucumber in a horizontal row on one side of the rice. Carefully close the bazooka.

10. Lay a piece of nori, shiny side down, on the sushi mat. Turn the plunger 5 times, then firmly press to release the roll onto one end of the nori. Tightly roll the nori around the rice to completely encase the roll. Transfer the roll to a cutting board. Rub a knife

on a damp paper towel before slicing the roll crosswise into 6 equal pieces. Repeat with the remaining ingredients to make another roll.

11. Assemble the board: Place the prawn crackers, musubi, and California rolls in the center of a turntable. Arrange the pan-fried dumplings, garlic edamame, scallion pancakes, dragonfruit, pineapple cakes, probiotic yogurt drinks, mochi, mujigae-tteok, Hello Panda cookies, Choco pies, Cara Cara and Mandarin oranges, and Asian pears around the edges.

12. Enjoy!

Sweet Potato Pie Smoothie

Ingredients

for 1 serving

• ⅓ cup ice (50 g)

• ¾ cup sweet potato (170 g), steamed

• 2 medjool dates, pitted, plus more, chopped, for topping

• ½ cup frozen riced cauliflower (150 g)

• 1 teaspoon maca powder

• ¼ teaspoon ground tumeric

• ¼ teaspoon ground cinnamon, plus more for topping

• 1 cup nondairy milk (240 mL), milk of your choice

Preparation

1. Combine the ice, sweet potato, dates, riced cauliflower, maca powder, turmeric, cinnamon, and

nondairy milk in a high-powered blender. Blend on high speed for 1–2 minutes, until completely smooth.

2. Pour the smoothie into a glass and top with a sprinkle of cinnamon and chopped dates.

3. Enjoy!

4. Don't let a good recipe slip away. Download the Tasty app and save your favorites for easy access.

Instant Pot Arroz Doce (Portuguese Sweet Rice)

Ingredients

for 10 servings

• 2 cups water (480 mL)

• 1 cup short grain rice (200 g)

• 2 cups whole milk (480 mL), warmed

• ½ cup sugar (100 g)

• 1 fresh lemon rind

• cinnamon, to taste

• 2 whole eggs, beaten

Preparation

1. Cook rice and water on a porridge setting for 20 mins using the 'quick release' setting. Then, turn on the saute feature, add milk, lemon rind, and sugar, and mix continuously for 20 minutes as mixture thickens.

2. Turn off the Instant Pot, then add eggs, mixing quickly to prevent scrambling. Remove lemon rind.

3. Pour into a serving dish and garnish with cinnamon in a criss-cross pattern. Let settle slightly.

4. Serve.

Chickpea Buddha Bowl

Ingredients

for 4 servings

Spiced Chickpeas

• 2 cans chickpeas, drained, rinsed, and patted dry

• 1 tablespoon olive oil

• 1 teaspoon McCormick® Himalayan Pink Salt with Black Pepper and Garlic

• ¼ teaspoon cumin

- ½ teaspoon paprika

- ½ teaspoon ground coriander

Garlic Herb Rice

- 1 cup jasmine rice (200 g)

- 1 teaspoon kosher salt

- 1 teaspoon Gourmet Gardens™ Garlic Paste

- 1 tablespoon Gourmet Garden™ Cilantro

- 1 tablespoon Gourmet Garden™ Parsley

Stewed Greens

- 1 tablespoon olive oil

- 2 large shallots, cut into ¼-inch (6 mm) rings

- 1 teaspoon Gourmet Garden™ Garlic Paste

* 2 large bunches hearty greens, (such as Swiss chard, kale, or mustard greens), stemmed and cut into ribbons

* ⅓ cup vegetable stock (80 mL)

* ½ teaspoon McCormick® Himalayan Pink Salt with Black Pepper and Garlic

Garlic Black Pepper Yogurt

* 1 cup full fat greek yogurt (245 g)

* ½ teaspoon Gourmet Garden™ Garlic Paste

* ½ teaspoon kosher salt, plus more to taste

* ½ teaspoon black pepper, plus more to taste

* water, as needed

For Serving

* 4 oz crumbled feta cheese (115 g)

• shaved radish, such as watermelon, breakfast, or black

• pickled red onion

• Gourmet Garden™ Cilantro

• Gourmet Garden™ Parsley

Preparation

1. Make the spiced chickpeas: Preheat the oven to 400°F (200°C).

2. In a large bowl, combine the chickpeas, olive oil, McCormick® Himalayan Pink Salt with Black Pepper and Garlic, paprika, cumin and coriander, and toss to coat.

3. Spread the chickpeas on a nonstick baking sheet and bake until crispy, about 20 minutes.

4. Make the garlic herb rice: Add the rice, salt, Gourmet Garden™ Garlic Paste, Gourmet Garden™ Cilantro, and Gourmet Garden™ Parsley to a medium pot. Add water and cook the rice according to the package instructions.

5. Make the stewed greens: In a large, high-walled skillet, heat the olive oil over medium heat. Add the shallots and cook for about 10 minutes, until soft and translucent. The shallots should start to develop some color, but shouldn't brown. Add the Gourmet Garden™ Garlic Paste, and cook until fragrant, about 1 minute. Add the greens, vegetable stock and McCormick® Himalayan Pink Salt with Black Pepper and Garlic, and gently stir to combine. Cover and cook, stirring occasionally, until the greens are wilted and soft, 5–7 minutes. Remove the pan from the heat, leaving the lid on to keep warm.

6. Make the garlic black pepper yogurt: In a medium bowl, whisk together the yogurt, Gourmet Garden™ Garlic Paste, salt, and pepper. Add a splash of water at a time and whisk to incorporate until the yogurt sauce is thin enough to drizzle. Season with more salt and pepper to taste.

7. Assemble the buddha bowls: Divide the rice evenly between 4 bowls. Top with the stewed greens, chickpeas, feta cheese, radish and pickled red onions. Drizzle the yogurt sauce over each bowl, then garnish with Gourmet Garden™ Parsley and Gourmet Garden™ Cilantro. Serve immediately.

8. Enjoy!

White Rice

Ingredients

for 4 servings

- 1 cup long grain rice (200 g)
- 1 ¾ cups water (420 mL)
- 1 pinch salt

Preparation

1. Rinse the rice in a sieve three times, or until the water runs clear.

2. Add the water and salt to a saucepan and bring to a boil over high heat.

3. Add the rice and stir, letting the water come to a boil again.

4. Place the lid on the saucepan and lower the heat to a simmer. Simmer for 18 minutes.

5. Turn off the heat and let the rice steam for 5 minutes.

6. Fluff the rice with a fork.

7. Enjoy!

Easy & Healthy Fried Rice

Ingredients

for 4 servings

• 2 tablespoons sesame oil

• 3 cloves garlic, minced

• 2 chicken breasts, diced

- salt, to taste

- pepper, to taste

- 1 cup carrot (120 g), diced

- 1 cup broccoli floret (175 g)

- 2 cups brown rice (400 g), cooked

- ½ cup frozen peas (75 g)

- 3 tablespoons low sodium soy sauce

Preparation

1. Heat sesame oil in a skillet, and cook garlic until softened.

2. Add the chicken, salt, and pepper, and sauté for 5 minutes.

3. Add the carrots and broccoli, and sauté until tender.

4. Add the rice, soy sauce, and peas, and mix thoroughly.

5. Enjoy!

Cilantro Lime Chicken & Veggie Rice Meal Prep

Ingredients

for 4 servings

• oil, of your preference, to taste

• 1 lb boneless, skinless chicken breast (455 g), cubed

• salt, to taste

• pepper, to taste

• 1 lime, juiced

- ⅓ cup fresh cilantro (15 g), minced

- 1 red bell pepper, diced

- ½ red onion, diced

- 2 cloves garlic, minced

- 1 bag riced cauliflower

- 1 cup corn (175 g), steamed

- ½ teaspoon chili powder, optional

- 1 can black beans, rinsed and drained, optional

- lime, cut into wedges, optional

Preparation

1. Heat preferred cooking oil in a large skillet over medium-high heat. Add chicken, season with salt and pepper, and cook until cooked through and no longer pink.

2. Add lime juice and cilantro. Stir to combine. Remove chicken from pan, place on a plate, and set aside.

3. Add a little more oil to pan if needed, then add red onion, bell pepper, and garlic. Stir to combine. Allow to cook until onion begins to turn transparent, stirring occasionally.

4. Add riced cauliflower, corn, and chili powder. Cook until cauliflower is soft and remove from heat.

5. Distribute black beans, chicken, and cauliflower mixture evenly between 4 containers. Top with a wedge of lime.

6. This meal prep can be refrigerated for up to 4 days.

7. Enjoy!

Orange Cauliflower "Chicken"

Ingredients

for 4 servings

• nonstick cooking spray, for greasing

• 2 cups non dairy milk (480 mL)

• 2 cups all purpose flour (250 g)

• 2 teaspoons kosher salt

• 1 cauliflower, cut into 1 1/2 inch (3 cm) florets

• 1 tablespoon canola oil

• 3 cloves garlic, minced

- 1 piece fresh ginger, minced

- ¼ teaspoon red pepper flakes

- ½ cup orange juice (120 mL)

- ½ cup brown sugar (100 g)

- ¼ cup distilled white vinegar (60 mL)

- ¼ cup soy sauce (60 mL)

- 2 tablespoons cornstarch

- 2 tablespoons cold water

- 1 teaspoon sesame oil

- white rice, for serving

- 3 scallions, thinly sliced, for garnish

Preparation

1. Preheat the oven to 450°F (230°C). Line a baking sheet with parchment paper and grease with nonstick spray.

2. In a medium bowl, whisk together the non-dairy milk, flour, and salt.

3. One at a time, dip each cauliflower floret in the batter to coat, letting any excess batter drip off. Arrange the battered cauliflower on the prepared baking sheet, making sure they aren't touching one another. Lightly spray with cooking spray.

4. Bake for 30–35 minutes, until the coating is crispy and beginning to brown.

5. While the cauliflower is baking, make the sauce: Heat the canola oil in a medium skillet over medium heat. When the oil is shimmering, add the garlic, ginger, and red pepper flakes. Cook for 2–3

minutes, until fragrant, stirring frequently to prevent burning.

6. Add the orange juice, brown sugar, vinegar, and soy sauce. Cook for 2–3 minutes, until the brown sugar is dissolved and the mixture begins to simmer.

7. In a small bowl, stir together the cornstarch and cold water with a fork.

8. Add the slurry to the sauce, stirring to combine. Simmer for another 2 minutes, until the sauce thickens. Mix in the sesame oil, then transfer the sauce to a large bowl.

9. Toss the hot cauliflower florets in the sauce until well coated.

10. Serve the cauliflower over rice and garnish with the scallions.

11. Enjoy!

One-pan Chicken Sausage & Veggies

Ingredients

for 4 servings

• 1 zucchini, sliced

• 1 yellow squash, sliced

• 1 tablespoon olive oil

• ¼ teaspoon salt

• ¼ teaspoon pepper

• ¼ teaspoon garlic powder

• 4 chicken sausages, fully cooked, sliced

• 4 cups wild rice (920 g), cooked, to serve

Preparation

1. Preheat the oven to 400°F (200°C).

2. Place the squash and zucchini on a baking sheet. Evenly coat with olive oil, salt, pepper, and garlic powder.

3. Push the squash and zucchini to the sides and place the chicken sausage in the middle.

4. Bake for 15 minutes, or until the zucchini and squash are tender.

5. Serve with wild rice. Eat immediately or refrigerate in airtight container up to 3-4 days.

6. Enjoy!

Chinese Takeout-style Tofu And Broccoli

Ingredients

for 4 servings

• 14 oz firm tofu

• 1 teaspoon vegetable oil

• 1 ½ teaspoons sesame oil, divided

• 3 cups broccoli florets

• 3 tablespoons vegetable broth

• 2 garlic cloves, minced

• 1 teaspoon grated ginger

• ¼ cup soy sauce

• 2 tablespoons agave syrup

• 1 tablespoon rice vinegar

• 1 tablespoon cornstarch, mixed with 1 tablespoon water

• $1\frac{1}{2}$ teaspoon toasted sesame seeds, plus more for serving

• cooked white rice, for serving

• sliced scallions, for serving

Preparation

1. Wrap the tofu in 2 layers of paper towels and place on a plate. Put another plate on top of the tofu to weigh it down and microwave for 2-3 minutes, or until drained.

2. After microwaving, carefully unwrap the tofu and slice into ½-1 inch cubes. Pat each cube dry.

3. In a large nonstick skillet, heat the vegetable oil and 1 teaspoon of sesame oil over medium-high heat. Once the oil is hot, add the tofu and cook on

all sides until golden brown, 2-4 minutes per side, then remove from the pan and set aside.

4. Add broccoli to the hot pan with the vegetable broth. Cover and reduce the heat to medium-low. Steam for 5 minutes.

5. Remove the lid and increase the heat to medium-high.

6. Add the garlic, ginger, and remaining ½ teaspoon of sesame oil. Stir until softened.

7. Add the soy sauce, agave, rice vinegar, and cornstarch slurry. Stir until thickened to your desired consistency. Add the sesame seeds and stir to incorporate.

8. Return the tofu to the pan and toss to coat in the sauce.

9. Serve over white rice and garnish with scallions and sesame seeds.

10. Enjoy!

Philadelphia Roll

Ingredients

for 4 servings

• 2 cups sushi rice (460 g)

• ¼ cup seasoned rice vinegar (60 mL)

• 4 half sheets sushi grade nori

• 4 oz smoked salmon (115 g)

• 4 oz cream cheese (115 g), cut into matchsticks

• 1 small cucumber, cut into matchsticks

Preparation

1. Season the sushi rice with the rice vinegar, fanning and stirring until room temperature.

2. On the rolling mat place one sheet of nori with the rough side facing upwards.

3. Wet your hands and grab a handful of rice and place it on the nori. Spread the rice evenly throughout the nori without smushing the rice down.

4. Arrange, in a horizontal row 1 inch (2 cm) from the bottom, smoked salmon, cream cheese, and cucumber.

5. Grabbing both nori and the mat, roll the mat over the filling so the extra space at the bottom touches the other side, squeezing down to make a nice tight

roll. Squeeze down along the way to keep the roll from holding its shape.

6. Transfer the roll onto a cutting board. Rub a knife on a damp paper towel before slicing the roll into six equal portions.

7. Enjoy!

Beef Broccoli-Stuffed Rice Triangles

Ingredients

for 12 servings

Rice

• 3 cups japanese short grain rice (600 g)

• 3 cups water (720 mL)

Stir Fry Sauce

- ½ cup soy sauce (120 mL)

- ¼ cup honey (85 g)

- ½ teaspoon ginger, minced

- 1 clove garlic, minced

Filling

- 1 tablespoon vegetable oil

- ½ lb boneless round steak (225 g), diced

- ½ teaspoon salt

- ½ teaspoon pepper

- ½ small yellow onion, finely chopped

- 1 cup broccoli (150 g), finely chopped

- 1 tablespoon cornstarch

- 1 tablespoon water

- ½ tablespoon sesame seeds

- 2 tablespoons vegetable oil

- ½ cup soy sauce (120 mL)

- scallion, thinly sliced, for garnish

Preparation

1. Make the rice: Wash the rice in a medium bowl of water, draining and refilling until the water is clear. Pour the washed rice into a large pot and add 3 cups (720 ml) of fresh water. Let soak for 30 minutes.

2. Place the rice on the stove over medium-high heat and bring to a boil. Cover, reduce the heat to low, and simmer for 12 minutes, or until all of the water is absorbed by the rice. Turn off the heat and let the rice rest with the lid on for 10 minutes, then fluff the rice and set aside until ready to use.

3. Make the stir fry sauce: In a liquid measuring cup or medium bowl, combine the soy sauce, honey, ginger, and garlic. Whisk to combine.

4. Make the filling: Heat the vegetable oil in a medium pan over medium heat. Add the beef, salt, and pepper and cook until the meat is browned and cooked all the way through, 3-4 minutes. Remove the beef from the pan.

5. Add the onion and broccoli to the same pan. Cook for 2-3 minutes, until slightly tender. Add the stir fry sauce. Combine the cornstarch and water in a small bowl and stir until cornstarch dissolves. Pour into the pan. Cook for 2-3 minutes more, or until the sauce is thick and the broccoli is tender.

6. Return the beef to the pan, add the sesame seeds, and stir until thoroughly combined. Remove the pan from the heat.

7. Line a 5-inch (13 cm) diameter bowl with plastic wrap. Scoop two tablespoons of rice into the bowl and use the back of a spoon (or your fingers) to flatten in an even layer against the inside of the bowl.

8. Add a ½ tablespoon of filling and top it off with a little more rice. Use the plastic wrap to mold the rice around the filling. Unwrap and use your hands to shape the rice into a triangle. Repeat with the remaining rice and filling.

9. In a medium pan, heat the vegetable oil over medium-high heat. Add 2-3 rice triangles to the pan and fry on each side for 1-2 minutes, or until the rice is crispy and starting to turn golden brown.

10. Brush soy sauce on all sides of the triangles and fry each side for another 1-2 minutes, or until dark golden brown. Repeat with the remaining triangles.

11. Sprinkle the rice triangles with scallions, then serve.

12. Enjoy!

Asian Chicken Chopped Salad

Ingredients

for 6 servings

• 2 chicken breasts

Marinade

• 2 tablespoons soy sauce

• 1 teaspoon sesame oil

• ½ teaspoon pepper

- ½ teaspoon red pepper flakes

- 1 garlic clove, sliced

- 1 tablespoon ginger, chopped

Dressing

- ¼ cup rice vinegar (60 mL)

- 1 tablespoon sesame oil

- 1 tablespoon soy sauce

- 1 tablespoon sugar

- 1 garlic clove, grated

- 1 teaspoon ginger, grated

Salad

- 2 romaine lettuces, chopped

- 1 cup red cabbage (100 g)

- ½ cup carrots (55 g), grated

- ¼ cup green onion (25 g), chopped

- ¼ cup cilantro (10 g), chopped

- ¼ cup almond slice (25 g)

- ¼ cup fried wonton chip (20 g)

Preparation

1. In a large bowl, combine marinade ingredients.

2. Add chicken into the bowl, coat the chicken, and marinate for 30 minutes in the fridge.

3. Fully cook chicken.

4. Cut into cubes.

5. In a mason jar, combine **Ingredients** for the dressing. Shake and set aside.

6. Prep the salad. Add all of the salad **Ingredients** into a large bowl and add the cubed chicken and dressing. Toss.

7. Enjoy!

California Roll

Ingredients

for 4 servings

• 2 cups sushi rice (460 g), cooked

• ¼ cup seasoned rice vinegar (60 mL)

• 4 half sheets sushi grade nori

• 1 teaspoon sesame seed, optional

• 8 pieces imitation crab

• 1 small cucumber, cut into matchsticks

• 1 avocado, thinly sliced

Preparation

1. Season the sushi rice with the rice vinegar, fanning and stirring until room temperature.

2. On a rolling mat, place one sheet of nori with the rough side facing upwards.

3. Wet your hands and grab a handful of rice and place it on the nori. Spread the rice evenly throughout the nori without mashing the rice down. Season rice with a pinch of sesame seeds, if using, then flip it over so the nori is facing upwards.

4. Arrange, in a horizontal row 1 inch (2.5 cm) from the bottom, the crab followed by a row of avocado and a row of cucumber.

5. Grabbing both nori and the mat, roll the mat over the filling so the extra space at the bottom touches the other side, squeezing down to make a nice tight roll. Squeeze down along the way to keep the roll from holding its shape.

6. Transfer the roll onto a cutting board. Rub a knife on a damp paper towel before slicing the roll into six equal portions.

7. Enjoy!

Rice Noodle Pancakes With Chili Sauce

Ingredients

for 5 pancakes

Sweet Chili Sauce

- ¾ cup water (180 mL)

- ¼ cup vinegar (60 mL)

- ½ cup sugar (100 g)

- ½ tablespoon salt

- 3 cloves garlic

- 2 serrano peppers, deseeded

Cornstarch Slurry

- 1 tablespoon cornstarch

- 2 tablespoons water

Rice Noodle Pancake

- 2 servings rice noodle

- 5 cups water (1 ¼ L), boiling

- 1 cup shredded carrots (110 g)

- ½ cup scallion (50 g), chopped

- 1 teaspoon grated ginger

- 1 tablespoon sesame oil

- 2 eggs, beaten

Preparation

1. In a blender or food processor, blend all of the sweet chili sauce ingredients together.

2. Pour into a saucepan and bring to a boil. Add the cornstarch slurry (dissolve 1 Tbsp. of cornstarch in 2 Tbsp. of water), stir and remove from heat. Set aside until ready to use.

3. Place a colander over a large mixing bowl. Add the rice noodles, pour the boiling water over and let it sit and soften for 10 minutes.

4. Drain, discard water and add the noodles to mixing bowl.

5. Using a pair of kitchen scissors, cut the noodles so they are easier to manage.

6. Add the carrots, scallions, ginger, sesame oil, beaten eggs. Mix well.

7. Grab a handful of noodles and place into your heated pan.

8. Using your spatula, flatten the noodles. Pan-fry until both sides are golden brown and crispy.

9. Serve with the sweet chili sauce.

10. Enjoy!

Cauliflower "Meat" Burrito Bowl

Ingredients

for 4 bowls

- 1 medium head cauliflower, washed

- 5 oz mushroom (140 g), such as baby bella, cleaned and quartered

- 1 ½ tablespoons olive oil

- 1 medium yellow onion, minced

- 2 cloves garlic, minced

- 2 teaspoons ground cumin

- 1 ½ teaspoons smoked paprika

- 2 tablespoons chili powder

- 2 tablespoons soy sauce

• salt, to taste

• pepper, to taste

• rice, cooked

• corn

• black bean

• avocado, sliced

• pico de gallo

• lime wedge

• fresh cilantro

Preparation

1. Cut the cauliflower in half and break it into small florets.

2. Place the florets in a food processor and pulse until they break down to rice-size pieces. Remove from the processor and set aside.

3. Add the mushrooms to the food processor and pulse until broken down to rice-size pieces.

4. Heat the olive oil in a large skillet over medium heat. Add the onion and garlic to the pan and cook for about 4 minutes, until fragrant and the onion is translucent.

5. Add the cauliflower, mushrooms, cumin, smoked paprika, chili powder, soy sauce, salt, and pepper and stir. Cook for about 10 minutes, until the cauliflower and mushroom mixture is tender and the water released from the mushrooms has evaporated.

6. Add the rice to a bowl and top with cauliflower "meat" and your favorite toppings. Serve with a lime wedge and garnish with cilantro.

7. If you have leftovers, the cauliflower "meat" will keep refrigerated in an airtight container for about 2 days.

8. Enjoy!

Buddha Bowl Meal Prep

Ingredients

for 4 servings

Chickpea Bowl

- 1 tablespoon oil

- 16 oz chickpeas (455 g), 1 can, drained and rinsed

- 1 teaspoon salt

- 1 teaspoon cumin

- ½ teaspoon garlic powder

- ½ teaspoon turmeric

- 1 teaspoon red pepper flakes

- 2 sweet potatoes

- oil, to taste

- salt, to taste

- pepper, to taste

- 1 cup quinoa (170 g), cooked

- 1 cup mixed greens (40 g)

- ½ avocado, sliced

- 1 tablespoon pumpkin seeds

Sauce

- 2 tablespoons hummus

- 1 tablespoon water

- ½ lemon, juiced

Tofu Bowl

- ½ package extra firm tofu, sliced in thirds

- ½ teaspoon ginger powder

- ½ teaspoon garlic powder

- salt, to taste

- pepper, to taste

- 2 cups broccoli floret (300 g)

- oil, to taste

- 1 cup brown rice (230 g), cooked

- ½ cup edamame (75 g)

- ½ cup shredded carrot (55 g)

- 2 teaspoons sesame seed

Sauce

- 2 tablespoons soy sauce

- 1 tablespoon sesame oil

- 1 teaspoon honey

- ½ teaspoon sriracha

Preparation

1. Preheat oven to 450°F (230°C).

2. Heat olive oil in a skillet over medium heat. Add chickpeas, salt, pepper, cumin, garlic powder,

turmeric, and chili flakes, and stir until toasted. Remove from pan.

3. Heat sesame oil in a skillet over medium heat. Add tofu, and sprinkle with ginger powder, garlic powder, salt, and pepper. Sear until a golden crust forms, then flip and do the same for the other side. Set aside.

4. On a baking sheet, toss sweet potatoes and broccoli in oil, salt, and pepper. Bake for 30 minutes.

5. In a bowl, combine ingredients for each sauce. Divide into 4 small tupperware containers.

6. To build the bowls, fill four tupperwares half with quinoa, half with brown rice. Layer the ingredients of each bowl on top.

7. When ready to eat, pour on dressing.

8. Enjoy!

Shrimp Tempura Rice Burger

Ingredients

for 3 servings

Tempura

• 1 egg

• 1 cup flour (120 g)

• ½ cup cold water (100 mL)

• flour, to cook

• 6 shrimps

• oil, to cook

Mayonnaise Sauce

- 3 tablespoons mayonnaise

- 1 tablespoon ketchup

- ½ tablespoon honey

- 1 teaspoon white vinegar

- 1 ¼ cups rice (300 g), cooked

- 2 tablespoons sesame oil, to cook

- green leaf lettuce, to taste

Preparation

1. Whisk the egg in a small bowl. Add 120 grams (1 cup) of flour and water. Whisk to combine. Cover with plastic wrap and transfer to the refrigerator.

2. Add flour to a shallow dish. Dip each shrimp in the flour, shaking off any excess.

3. Dip the floured shrimp into the batter.

4. Heat oil in a pot to 350°F (180°C).

5. Fry the shrimp until they float to the top and become golden brown in color. Use a slotted spoon to transfer the shrimp to a paper towel-lined plate to drain.

6. For the mayonnaise sauce, combine mayonnaise, ketchup, honey, and vinegar.

7. Line a ramekin with plastic wrap, and mold ¼ of the rice into a patty. Repeat until you have 6 rice "buns."

8. Heat a pan over medium-high heat and add a splash of sesame oil. Add the rice "buns" and cook until the outside is crispy, about 5 minutes.

9. Top the rice "bun" with a piece of green leaf lettuce, fried shrimps, mayonnaise sauce, and top

with another rice "bun." Repeat with remaining ingredients.

10. Enjoy!

Watermelon "Poke" Bowl

Ingredients

for 4 servings

• 1 mini watermelon, sliced

• 6 tablespoons soy sauce

• 2 teaspoons rice vinegar

• 1 tablespoon sesame oil

• 1 lime, juiced

- 1 tablespoon agave nectar

- 2 scallions, minced

- 2 tablespoons fresh ginger, minced

- 2 tablespoons white sesame seeds, toasted

- 1 teaspoon red chile flakes

- 1 medium cucumber

- 6 tablespoons mayonnaise

- 2 tablespoons sriracha

- white rice, cooked, for serving

- avocado, sliced, for serving

- shelled edamame, for serving

- nori sheet, for serving

- pickled ginger, for serving

• fresh cilantro, for serving

• peanut, crushed, for serving

• black sesame seed, for garnish, optional

Preparation

1. Using a sharp knife, cut around the watermelon slices rind to remove, then dice into 1-inch (2 cm) cubes.

2. Transfer 4 cups (600 g) to a medium bowl, reserving the rest for another use.

3. In a small bowl, combine the soy sauce, rice vinegar, sesame oil, lime juice, agave, scallions, ginger, white sesame seeds, and chile flakes. Mix well.

4. Pour the marinade over the watermelon cubes and stir. Cover the bowl with plastic wrap and let marinate in the fridge for 1 hour.

5. Slice the cucumber into thin half moons and set aside.

6. In a small bowl, combine the mayo and Sriracha.

7. To assemble the poke bowls, start with rice as a base and top with cucumbers, avocado, edamame, nori, pickled ginger, Sriracha mayo, cilantro, and crushed peanuts.

8. Add a scoop of the marinated watermelon and use the marinade as a dressing to drizzle over the bowl.

9. Garnish with black sesame seeds, if desired.

10. Enjoy!

Spring Vegetable Chowder

Ingredients

for 6 servings

• ¼ cup olive oil (60 mL), divided, plus more for drizzling

• 20 oz riced cauliflower (565 g)

• 5 oz leeks (140 g), tough green ends removed, cut into half-moons and rinsed

• 5 cloves garlic, smashed

• 1 tablespoon kosher salt, plus 2 teaspoons, divided, plus more to taste

• 4 cups vegetable stock (960 mL)

• 2 cups non-dairy milk (480 mL), plus more to taste, divided

• 10 oz asparagus (285 g), woody stems removed, cut into 1/2-in (1 1/4-cm) pieces

• 1 ½ cups frozen english peas (170 g)

• 1 lemon, zested

• ¼ cup thinly sliced fresh basil (10 g), plus more for garnish

• 1 ½ lb medium red potatoes (680 g), cut into 1/2 in (1 1/4 cm) cubes

• cold water, as needed

• 2 tablespoons fresh lemon juice

• freshly ground black pepper, for garnish

Preparation

1. In a large pot, heat 2 tablespoons of olive oil over medium heat. Once the oil is shimmering, add the riced cauliflower, leeks, garlic, and 1 teaspoon of

salt. Sauté for 2 minutes, until the leeks just begin to soften.

2. Pour in the vegetable stock and 2 cups (480 ml) of non-dairy milk. Increase the heat to medium-high and bring to a boil. Reduce the heat to medium, cover, and simmer for 15-20 minutes, until the cauliflower is completely broken down and tender.

3. Meanwhile, in a large pan, heat 2 tablespoons of olive oil over medium heat. Add the asparagus, peas, and 1 teaspoon of salt. Sauté for 2 minutes, until the vegetables are bright green with some crunch. Remove the pan from the heat and stir in the lemon zest and basil. Transfer to a bowl and set aside.

4. Wipe out the pan and add the potatoes and enough cold water to cover by 1 inch (1 ¼ cm).

Season with 1 tablespoon of salt. Bring to a boil. Once boiling, reduce the heat to medium-low and simmer for 8-10 minutes, until the potatoes are easily pierced with a fork but not mushy. Drain and set aside.

5. Remove the pot with the cauliflower from the heat. Blend with an immersion blender until completely smooth and creamy. Add up to 1 cup (240 ml) non-dairy milk or water if needed to thin to your desired consistency.

6. Stir in the reserved asparagus, peas, potatoes, and the lemon juice. Season to taste with salt.

7. Ladle into bowls and garnish with fresh basil, a drizzle of olive oil, and freshly ground black pepper.

8. Enjoy!

Za'atar Chicken And Rice Pilaf

Ingredients

for 4 servings

• 5 lb whole chicken (2 ¼ kg)

Brine

• 1 tablespoon whole black peppercorn

• 1 tablespoon fennel seeds

• 1 tablespoon coriander seed

• 4 qt water (4 L), divided

• 4 sprigs fresh oregano

• 4 sprigs fresh thyme

• 3 dried bay leaves

• ½ cup kosher salt (120 g)

- ½ cup dark brown sugar (110 g), packed

- ¼ cup soy sauce (60 mL), or tamari

Chicken Seasoning

- 1 oz lemon peel (30 g), chopped

- 1 oz garlic (30 g), chopped

- 3 tablespoons canola oil, or other neutral oil

- 8 tablespoons unsalted butter, cut into

- 1 teaspoon kosher salt

- 2 teaspoons za'atar

Rice Pilaf

- 2 cups chicken stock (480 mL)

- 1 tablespoon unsalted butter

- 2 garlics, halved lengthwise

- ½ cup fideo (75 g), broken vermicelli noodles

- 1 ½ cups white basmati rice (300 g)

- za'atar oil

- ¼ cup olive oil (60 mL)

- 1 ½ teaspoons za'atar

- ¼ teaspoon kosher salt

For Serving

- 2 tablespoons fresh flat-leaf parsley

- 1 lemon, cut into 8 wedges

Preparation

1. Spatchcock the chicken: Place the chicken, breast-side down, on a cutting board. Using a pair of kitchen shears or a very sharp knife, find the backbone of the chicken and cut up both sides to

remove. Remove any giblets remaining inside the chicken. Turn the chicken over and press down on the breastbone until the chicken lies flat.

2. Make the brine: In a small, dry pan, toast the peppercorns, fennel seeds, and coriander seeds until fragrant and starting to change color, 1-2 minutes.

3. Transfer the toasted spices to a large pot with 1 quart (1 liter) of water, the oregano, thyme, bay leaves, salt, brown sugar, and soy sauce. Bring to a boil over high heat, stirring to dissolve the sugar and salt, then let boil for 1 minute. Remove the pot from the heat. Transfer the brine to a large container. Cool the brine by adding the remaining water.

4. Place the chicken in the brine, cover the container, and chill in the refrigerator for at least 6 hours, or overnight.

5. Preheat the oven to 450°F (230°C). Place a wire rack or roasting rack on top of a baking sheet.

6. Make the chicken seasoning: In a food processor, combine the lemon peel, garlic, and canola oil. Process into a thick paste.

7. Remove the chicken from the brine and pat dry with paper towels. Use your fingers to carefully separate the skin from the breasts and thighs. Rub the lemon garlic paste over the bird, making sure to get some under the skin. Rub the softened butter underneath and over the skin. Season on both sides with the salt and za'atar. Place the chicken on the rack set over the baking sheet, breast-side up.

8. Roast the chicken for 40-50 minutes, until the breast meat reaches 145°F (63°C).

9. Roast until the thigh meat, near the bones, reaches 160°F (71°C). Remove from the oven and let rest for 5-10 minutes.

10. Meanwhile, make the rice pilaf: Place the rice in a fine-mesh sieve and rinse under running water until the water runs clear. Transfer the rice to a medium bowl and cover with water by 1 inch (2.5 cm). Soak for 10 minutes.

11. Add the chicken stock to a small pot and bring to a boil, then cover and reduce the heat to low so the stock stays warm.

12. In a large pot or pan over medium heat, combine the butter, garlic, and fideo. Cook, stirring constantly, until most of the noodles are golden brown, about 5 minutes.

13. Drain the rice once the noodles are toasted, then add to the pan and sauté until the rice is dry and coated with the butter, 2-3 minutes.

14. Add the hot chicken stock, then reduce the heat to low, cover, and cook until the noodles curl up, about 15 minutes. Fluff the pilaf with a fork, then cover again and let sit for at least 5 minutes before serving.

15. Make the za'atar oil: In a small bowl, mix together the olive oil, za'atar, and salt.

16. Carve the chicken, then arrange over the rice pilaf and spoon the za'atar oil over. Garnish with parsley and serve with lemon wedges.

17. Enjoy!

Vegan Black Rice Sushi Rolls

Ingredients

for 3 rolls

Sushi

- ⅓ cup organic tempeh (55 g), cut into thin strips

- ⅓ cup soy sauce (80 mL)

- 1 medium carrot, grated

- ¼ head purple cabbage, grated

- 3 sheets toasted nori

- black rice, cooked according to package directions, and cooled

- ½ cup avocado (75 g), thinly sliced lengthwise

- ⅓ cup english cucumber (50 g), seeded, cut into thin strips

- ⅓ cup cashews (45 g), coarsely chopped

- water, for sealing

Sesame Miso Sauce

- 3 tablespoons olive oil

- ¼ cup lime juice (60 mL)

- 3 tablespoons maple syrup

- 2 teaspoons white miso paste

- 2 teaspoons black sesame seeds

- 1 teaspoon fresh ginger, grated, optional

Special Equipment

- bamboo sushi mat, optional

Preparation

1. In a medium bowl, pour the soy sauce over the tempeh. Set aside to marinate for at least 25 minutes. While the tempeh marinates, prepare the rest of the ingredients.

2. Heat a medium nonstick pan over medium-high heat. Add the marinated tempeh strips. Cook for 1-2 minutes on each side, until golden brown and lightly charred. Remove from the pan and set aside to cool.

3. In a medium bowl, toss together the carrot and cabbage.

4. Build the sushi rolls: Lay a sheet of toasted nori, shiny side down, on the bamboo mat or clean work surface. Pat about ¼ of the rice evenly over the nori, leaving about a ½ inch (1 ¼ cm) of space at the top. Layer a few slices of avocado over the rice toward the bottom of the nori sheet. Top with a few pieces

of cucumber, some of the carrot-cabbage mixture, a couple of pieces of tempeh, and about 1 tablespoon of chopped cashews.

5. To close the sushi roll, brush a bit of water across the empty edge of the nori. Using both hands, roll the filled end of the nori sheet over onto itself, carefully tucking all of the ingredients inside. Continue rolling until the nori sheet covers the rice and seal with the damp edge. Repeat with remaining nori sheets and fillings.

6. With a sharp knife, cut each roll into 6-8 pieces, depending on preference. Pro tip: If you wet the knife before slicing, it will cut through the nori more cleanly. But be careful!

7. Make the sesame miso sauce: In a small bowl, combine the olive oil, lime juice, maple syrup, miso,

sesame seeds, and ginger, if using. Whisk to combine.

8. Serve the sushi rolls with the sauce for dipping.

9. Enjoy!

Weekday Meal-prep Chicken Teriyaki Stir-fry

Ingredients

for 4 servings

• 3 chicken breasts, cubed

• salt, to taste

• pepper, to taste

• 1 teaspoon garlic, crushed

• ½ cup soy sauce (118 mL)

- ⅓ cup honey (113 g)

- 1 ½ tablespoons sesame seed, more to garnish

- 1 onion, sliced

- 2 small bell peppers, thinly sliced

- 2 cups broccoli (500 g)

- 1 green onion, thinly sliced

- white rice, cooked

Preparation

1. In a pan, cook cut chicken over medium-high heat until almost done. Salt and pepper to taste.

2. Reduce heat to medium and stir in the crushed garlic.

3. Add in the soy sauce, honey, and 1 tablespoon of the sesame seeds. Stir until thickened.

4. Remove the chicken from the pan, leaving the sauce, and add the vegetables to the pan.

5. Cover the pan for several minutes and cook until the vegetables begin to soften, then remove the lid and stir until the sauce is thick again.

6. Split the rice, vegetables, and chicken evenly between 4 containers. Top with a sprinkle of sesame seeds and sliced green onion. Refrigerate for up to 4 days.

7. Enjoy!

Lentils and Rice With Caramelized Onions

Ingredients

for 4 servings

Lentils and Rice

- 1 tablespoon olive oil

- ½ medium red onion, diced

- 2 cloves garlic, minced

- 3 ½ cups water (840 mL)

- 1 cup green lentils (200 g)

- 1 teaspoon salt

- 1 cup long grain rice (200 g)

- ½ teaspoon ground cinnamon

- 1 teaspoon ground cumin

- 1 dried bay leaf

Caramelized Onions

- 1 tablespoon olive oil

• 1 medium red onion, thinly sliced

For Serving

• 1 bunch finely chopped fresh parsley

• 1 lemon, cut into wedges

• ½ cup greek yogurt (120 g)

Preparation

1. Make the lentils and rice: Heat the olive oil in a large pot with a lid over medium heat. Add the diced red onion and minced garlic and sauté until translucent, about 5 minutes.

2. Add the water, lentils, and salt and bring to a boil. Cover with the lid and simmer for 10 minutes.

3. Meanwhile, make the caramelized onions: Heat the olive oil in a large skillet over low heat. Add the sliced onion and cook, stirring frequently to prevent

burning, until completely soft, dark brown, and caramelized, 25–30 minutes.

4. Add the rice, cinnamon, cumin, and bay leaf to the pot with the lentils. Stir to combine. Cover again and cook for about 15 minutes, until the rice is tender.

5. Serve the lentils and rice topped with the caramelized onions and parsley, with lemon wedges and Greek yogurt alongside, if desired.

6. Enjoy!

One-Pot Enchilada Rice

Ingredients

for 4 servings

- 1 tablespoon oil

- 1 tablespoon minced garlic, minced

- ½ cup red onion (75 g), chopped

- 1 cup bell pepper (100 g), chopped

- 1 cup tomato (200 g), chopped

- 3 cups water (720 mL)

- 1 ½ cups rice (300 g)

- 1 cup black beans (170 g)

- 1 tablespoon fresh cilantro, chopped

- 1 cup tomato sauce (260 g)

- 1 teaspoon chili powder

- 1 teaspoon cumin

- 1 teaspoon salt

- 1 teaspoon pepper

- ½ cup shredded cheese (50 g), optional

- ½ avocado, cubed, for garnish

Preparation

1. Preheat oven to 400ºF (200ºC).

2. Put oil in a cast-iron skillet over medium heat. Add garlic and onion to skillet and stir until garlic is slightly golden and onion has softened.

3. Add pepper and sauté 2-3 minutes or until peppers have softened.

4. Add tomatoes and sauté 1 minute.

5. Remove sauteed vegetables and set aside.

6. Pour water into the skillet and wait for it to come to a boil.

7. Add rice and stir for 12-15 minutes until rice is fluffier but still slightly tender.

8. Make a circle in the center of the rice and add your sautéed vegetables and black beans to the skillet and mix.

9. Add cilantro, tomato sauce, chili powder, cumin, salt, and pepper, and stir.

10. Add cheese on top (optional).

11. Bake in a preheated oven for 20-25 minutes.

12. Allow to cool for 5 minutes.

13. Garnish with cilantro and avocado (optional).

14. Enjoy!

Slow Cooker Chicken Tikka Masala

Ingredients

for 4 servings

• 2 cups chicken (250 g)

• 1 tablespoon flour

• 2 teaspoons salt

• 1 tablespoon garam masala

• 1 tablespoon turmeric

• 1 tablespoon paprika

• 1 onion, chopped

• 4 cloves garlic, minced

• 2 green chiles, chopped

• ½ cup tomato (100 g), in their juices

• 2 tablespoons tomato puree

• ¾ cup plain yogurt (200 g)

Garnish

• rice

• coriander

Preparation

1. Place the chicken pieces in the slow cooker and coat well with the flour and salt.

2. Throw in the garam masala, turmeric, paprika, onions, garlic, chillies, chopped tomatoes and tomato puree and mix together.

3. Slow cook on high for 3 hours.

4. After 3 hours, stir in the plain yogurt. Serve with rice and top with chopped coriander.

5. Enjoy!

Cilantro Lime Chicken & Veggie Rice Meal Prep

Ingredients

for 4 servings

• oil, of your preference, to taste

• 1 lb boneless, skinless chicken breast (455 g), cubed

• salt, to taste

• pepper, to taste

• 1 lime, juiced

- ⅓ cup fresh cilantro (15 g), minced

- 1 red bell pepper, diced

- ½ red onion, diced

- 2 cloves garlic, minced

- 1 bag riced cauliflower

- 1 cup corn (175 g), steamed

- ½ teaspoon chili powder, optional

- 1 can black beans, rinsed and drained, optional

- lime, cut into wedges, optional

Preparation

1. Heat preferred cooking oil in a large skillet over medium-high heat. Add chicken, season with salt and pepper, and cook until cooked through and no longer pink.

2. Add lime juice and cilantro. Stir to combine. Remove chicken from pan, place on a plate, and set aside.

3. Add a little more oil to pan if needed, then add red onion, bell pepper, and garlic. Stir to combine. Allow to cook until onion begins to turn transparent, stirring occasionally.

4. Add riced cauliflower, corn, and chili powder. Cook until cauliflower is soft and remove from heat.

5. Distribute black beans, chicken, and cauliflower mixture evenly between 4 containers. Top with a wedge of lime.

6. This meal prep can be refrigerated for up to 4 days.

7. Enjoy!

Ghanaian Jollof Rice

Ingredients

for 6 servings

• 2 large yellow onions, roughly chopped

• ⅓ cup vegetable oil (80 mL), plus 2 tablespoons, divided

• 14 oz diced tomato (395 g), 2 cans

• 6 oz tomato paste (170 g), 1 can

• 1 habanero pepper

• 2 teaspoons curry powder

• 1 teaspoon garlic powder

• 1 teaspoon ground ginger

• ½ teaspoon mixed dried herbs

- 3 chicken bouillon cubes, crushed

- 2 ½ cups long grain rice (500 g), rinsed

- 1 cup frozen mixed vegetable (150 g)

- 1 ½ cups water (360 mL)

Preparation

1. Add onions and 2 tablespoons of oil to a blender and pulse until smooth. Transfer to a medium bowl.

2. Add the diced tomatoes, tomato paste, and habanero pepper to the blender, and pulse until smooth. Transfer to a separate medium bowl.

3. Heat the remaining ⅓ cup (80 ml) of oil in a large, heavy-bottomed pot over medium heat.

4. Once the oil is shimmering, add the onion puree and cook until the water has cooked out and the puree is starting to brown, about 10 minutes.

5. Stir in the tomato puree and add the curry powder, garlic powder, ginger, dried herbs, and crushed bouillon cubes. Cook for 20-30 minutes, stirring occasionally, until the stew has reduced by half and is deep red in color.

6. Add the rice, mixed vegetables, and water. Bring to a boil, then reduce the heat to low and cover the pot with foil and a lid. Simmer for another 30 minutes, until the rice is cooked through and the liquid is absorbed.

7. Enjoy!

One-Pan Miso Honey Salmon For Two

Ingredients

for 2 servings

• 2 tablespoons white miso paste

• 2 tablespoons honey

• 1 tablespoon rice vinegar

• 1 teaspoon garlic, minced

• 1 teaspoon ginger, grated

• pepper, to taste

• 3 oz salmon (85 g), 2 fillets

• ½ bunch asparagus, trimmed

• 1 large baby bok choy, halved lengthwise

• olive oil, to taste

• salt, to taste

• brown rice, cooked, for serving, optional

• sesame seed, for garnish

Preparation

1. Preheat the oven to 400°F (200°C) and line a baking sheet with parchment paper.

2. In a small bowl, combine the miso paste, honey, rice vinegar, garlic, ginger, and pepper. Whisk until smooth.

3. Place the salmon fillets skin-side down in the center of the prepared baking sheet and brush generously with the miso-honey sauce.

4. Lay the asparagus on one side of the salmon and the baby bok choy on the other side. Drizzle the vegetables with olive oil and season with salt and pepper. Rub the vegetables until evenly coated.

5. Bake for 10-12 minutes, or until the salmon is cooked to your liking.

6. Divide the vegetables and salmon between serving plates, with rice alongside if desired. Garnish the salmon with sesame seeds and serve immediately.

7. Enjoy!

Thai Coconut Vegetable Curry

Ingredients

for 8 servings

• 1 tablespoon coconut oil

• 1 red onion, thinly sliced

• 1 medium jalapeno, seeded and finely chopped

• 3 cloves garlic, minced

- 1 orange bell pepper, seeded and cut into thin strips

- 1 large eggplant, ends trimmed, diced

- 3 tablespoons red curry paste

- 1 tablespoon brown sugar

- 13.5 oz light coconut milk (400 mL)

- 28 oz diced tomatoes (790 g)

- 13.5 oz chickpeas (380 g), drained and rinsed

- 5 oz baby spinach (140 g)

- ¼ cup chopped fresh cilantro (10 g)

- cooked brown rice, for serving

Preparation

1. Melt the coconut oil in a large, high-walled pan over medium heat. Add the onion and cook for 2

minutes, until just beginning to sweat. Add the jalapeño and garlic, and sauté for 1 minute, until just fragrant. Add the bell pepper and eggplant and cook for 3 minutes, until the eggplant begins to soften.

2. Add the curry paste and brown sugar and stir to coat the vegetables, making sure there are no large clumps of curry paste. Pour in the coconut milk and stir to combine until the milk is stained from the curry paste. Stir in the diced tomatoes and chickpeas and bring to a gentle simmer for 5 minutes.

3. Once the curry is simmering, add the spinach, half at a time, and stir until wilted. Remove the pan from the heat.

4. Garnish the curry with cilantro and serve over brown rice.

5. Nutrition Calories: 212 Total fat: 7 grams Sodium: 368 Total carbs: 34 grams Dietary fiber: 8 grams Sugars: 10 grams Protein: 7 grams

6. Enjoy!

One-pan Chicken Sausage & Veggies

Ingredients

for 4 servings

• 1 zucchini, sliced

• 1 yellow squash, sliced

• 1 tablespoon olive oil

• ¼ teaspoon salt

• ¼ teaspoon pepper

• ¼ teaspoon garlic powder

• 4 chicken sausages, fully cooked, sliced

• 4 cups wild rice (920 g), cooked, to serve

Preparation

1. Preheat the oven to 400°F (200°C).

2. Place the squash and zucchini on a baking sheet. Evenly coat with olive oil, salt, pepper, and garlic powder.

3. Push the squash and zucchini to the sides and place the chicken sausage in the middle.

4. Bake for 15 minutes, or until the zucchini and squash are tender.

5. Serve with wild rice. Eat immediately or refrigerate in airtight container up to 3-4 days.

6. Enjoy!

Kung Pao Cauliflower Bites

Ingredients

for 4 servings

Batter

• 1 cup all-purpose flour (125 g)

• 1 teaspoon baking soda

• 1 ½ cups soy milk (360 mL), or water

• 1 head cauliflower, cut into florets

Sauce

• ½ cup soy sauce (120 mL)

• ½ cup agave nectar (120 mL)

• 1 tablespoon sesame oil

• 1 tablespoon rice vinegar

• 2 cloves garlic, minced

• 2 teaspoons ginger

• 1 tablespoon cornstarch

• fresh chive, finely chopped, for serving

• sesame seed, for serving

• rice, cooked, for serving

Preparation

1. Preheat the oven to 450ºF (230ºC). Line a baking sheet with parchment paper.

2. In a large bowl, combine the flour, baking soda, and soy milk, and whisk until smooth.

3. Add the cauliflower florets to the batter and toss until fully coated.

4. Transfer the coated cauliflower to the baking sheet and bake for 10 minutes, or until the coating looks dry.

5. Meanwhile, in a medium saucepan over high heat, combine the soy sauce, agave, sesame oil, rice vinegar, garlic, ginger, and cornstarch, and stir until the mixture comes to a boil. Turn off the heat and let sit for 10 minutes to thicken.

6. Remove the cauliflower from the oven and transfer to a large bowl to cool for 5 minutes. Leave the oven on.

7. Add the sauce to the bowl and toss the cauliflower until completely coated, then return to a parchment-lined baking sheet and bake for another 10 minutes.

8. Top the cauliflower with chives and sesame seeds, and serve over rice, if desired.

9. Enjoy!

Healthy Veggie Curry With Garlic Naan

Ingredients

for 8 servings

Rice

• 2 cups white rice (400 g), rinsed

• 4 cups water (960 g)

• 1 tablespoon coconut oil, melted

• salt, to taste

Curry

• ¼ cup vegetable oil (60 mL), divided

• 2 small yellow onions, diced

• 2 cups idaho potato (450 g), cubed

• 1 tablespoon tomato paste

• 2 tablespoons fresh ginger, minced

• 3 cloves garlic, minced

• 1 ½ teaspoons garam masala

• 2 tablespoons curry powder

• 1 head cauliflower, cut into small florets

• 15 oz diced tomato (425 g), 1 can

• 15 oz chickpeas (425 g), 1 can, drained

• 1 ¼ cups water (360 mL)

• salt, to taste

• ¾ cup coconut milk (180 mL)

• 1 ¼ cups frozen peas (190 g)

Garlic Naan

• 2 cups all-purpose flour (250 g)

• 1 teaspoon salt

• 1 teaspoon baking powder

• 1 teaspoon sugar

• 2 tablespoons ghee, melted, divided, plus more as needed

• 4 tablespoons whole-fat yogurt

• 2 tablespoons skim milk

• 6 tablespoons water

• 1 clove garlic, minced

Preparation

1. In a medium pot, combine the rice, water, coconut oil, and salt. Bring to a boil, then cover and simmer over low heat for 15-20 minutes, until the water is absorbed. Once finished cooking, remove the rice from the heat and fluff.

2. Heat 3 tablespoons of vegetable oil in a large Dutch oven over medium-high heat until shimmering. Add the onions and potatoes and cook, stirring occasionally, until the onions are caramelized and potatoes are golden brown around the edges, about 10 minutes.

3. Reduce the heat to medium. Add the remaining tablespoon of oil, the tomato paste, ginger, and garlic. Cook, stirring constantly, until fragrant, about 30 seconds. Add the garam masala and curry powder and cook, stirring constantly, about 1 minute longer.

4. Add cauliflower and cook, stirring constantly, until the spices coat the florets, about 2 minutes longer.

5. Add the tomatoes, chickpeas, water, and salt and stir to combine. Increase the heat to medium-high and bring the mixture to a boil. Reduce the heat to medium. Simmer, stirring occasionally, until the vegetables are tender, 10-15 minutes.

6. Stir in the coconut milk and frozen peas. Cook until heated through, about 2 minutes longer. Remove from the heat.

7. Meanwhile, in a large bowl, stir together the flour, salt, baking powder, and sugar. Create a well in the middle of the dry **Ingredients** and pour in 1 tablespoon of melted ghee, the yogurt, skim milk, and a bit of the water. Mix until combined, adding

more water as needed until the dough comes together.

8. Transfer the dough to a lightly floured surface and knead until no longer sticky, then shape into a ball and divide into quarters. Roll out the dough portions to ¼ inch (6 mm) thick.

9. In a small bowl, combine the remaining tablespoon of melted ghee with the garlic.

10. Heat a bit of ghee in a medium nonstick pan over medium-high heat. Add a dough round and brush with the ghee and garlic mixture. Cook for 3-4 minutes, until the dough bubbles up and forms a nice brown crust, then flip and cook on the other side. Repeat with the remaining dough.

11. Serve the curry over the rice with the naan on the side.

12. Enjoy!

Tachin Joojeh

Ingredients

for 4 servings

Marinated Chicken

- 1 cup full fat greek yogurt (245 g)

- 1 tablespoon lemon zest

- 1 teaspoon garlic

- 1 tablespoon ground turmeric

- 1 tablespoon black pepper

- 1 teaspoon fresh ginger

- 1 tablespoon kosher salt

• 1 ½ lb boneless, skinless chicken breast (680 g)

Yogurt Rice

• 4 cups water (960 mL)

• 2 ¼ cups basmati rice (450 g), rinsed

• ¼ teaspoon saffron thread, optional

• 1 tablespoon warm water, optional

• ¾ cup plain full-fat greek yogurt (185 g)

• 2 large egg yolks

• 1 tablespoon ground turmeric

• ½ teaspoon ground cumin

• ½ teaspoon kosher salt

• ½ teaspoon black pepper

Chicken And Onions

- 2 tablespoons olive oil

- 1 medium white onion, sliced

- 1 teaspoon fresh ginger, minced

- 1 tablespoon garlic, minced

- 1 teaspoon ground cumin

- 1 teaspoon kosher salt

Assembly

- 2 tablespoons softened butter

- 3 tablespoons olive oil, divided

- ½ cup barberries (50 g), sultanas or currants

- 1 pinch kosher salt

Yogurt Sauce

- 1 cup plain full-fat greek yogurt (245 g)

- 1 tablespoon fresh mint leaf

- 1 tablespoon fresh parsley, chopped

- 1 teaspoon kosher salt

- ½ teaspoon black pepper

- ¼ teaspoon ground cumin

- 1 teaspoon fresh ginger, minced

- ½ teaspoon garlic, minced

- ½ teaspoon lemon zest

- ½ lemon, juiced

Preparation

1. Make the marinade: In a large bowl, mix together the yogurt, lemon zest, garlic, turmeric, pepper, ginger, and salt. Add the chicken and toss to coat. Cover the bowl with plastic wrap and marinate the

chicken in the refrigerator for at least 1 hour, or overnight.

2. Preheat the oven to 400°F (200°C).

3. Make the yogurt rice: Add the water to a medium pot and bring to a boil over high heat. Add the rice and simmer for 3 minutes. Drain the rice and rinse with cold water to stop the cooking process. The rice should be slightly translucent with a completely opaque center. Set aside to drain completely.

4. If using the saffron, combine with the warm water in a small bowl. Cover with plastic wrap or a lid and let bloom for about 5 minutes, until the water has cooled.

5. In a medium bowl, mix together the yogurt, egg yolks, turmeric, cumin, salt, pepper, and bloomed

saffron, if using, until bright orange-yellow. Add half of the rice and stir to incorporate. Set aside.

6. Cook the chicken and onions: Wipe the marinade off the chicken, then cut into bite-size pieces.

7. Heat the olive oil in a medium pan over medium heat. When the oil is shimmering, add the onion and cook until just translucent, about 5 minutes. Add the ginger, garlic, cumin, and salt. Cook for 1 minute, until the garlic and ginger are fragrant, then add the chicken and cook until just cooked through, about 7 minutes. Remove the pan from the heat.

8. Grease a 2½-quart ovenproof glass bowl or a 5-inch square casserole dish with the butter and 2 tablespoons of olive oil.

9. Add the yogurt rice to the prepared bowl and pack down with a spatula. Evenly distribute chicken

and onion mixture over the yogurt rice and pack down. Add the remaining cooked rice on top in an even layer. Cut a piece of parchment paper to cover the bowl and then wrap tightly with foil.

10. Bake for 45 minutes, until the rice on the bottom is crispy and browned.

11. Meanwhile, make the yogurt sauce: In a medium bowl, mix together the yogurt, mint, parsley, salt, pepper, cumin, ginger, garlic, lemon zest, and lemon juice.

12. In a small pan, heat the remaining tablespoon of olive oil over medium heat until shimmering. Add the barberries and sauté for 3 minutes, until warmed. Remove the pan from the heat and season with a pinch of salt.

13. To serve, carefully invert the bowl onto a serving platter or cutting board. If it does not release, take

a spatula and run it along the sides, then try again. Spoon some of the yogurt sauce over the top and sprinkle with the barberries. Serve with the remaining yogurt sauce alongside.

14. Enjoy!

Orange Glazed Meatballs and Veggies

Ingredients

for 4 servings

• ½ cup broccoli (125 g)

• 1 carrot

• ¼ onion

• olive oil

- salt, to taste

- pepper, to taste

Meatball

- 1 lb ground turkey (455 g), or ground chicken

- 1 egg

- ¼ cup panko breadcrumbs (15 g)

- 2 cloves garlic, minced

- 2 teaspoons ginger, grated

- 2 tablespoons green onion

- 2 tablespoons soy sauce

- salt, to taste

- pepper, to taste

Sauce

- ¾ cup orange marmalade (240 g)

- ¼ cup rice vinegar (60 mL)

- 1 teaspoon sesame oil

- 1 clove garlic, minced

- 1 teaspoon ginger, minced

- 1 teaspoon salt

- ½ teaspoon pepper

Preparation

1. Preheat oven to 475°F (240°C).

2. In a bowl, combine all ingredients for the meatballs. Mix until all ingredients are incorporated.

3. Using your hands or a spoon, roll a bit of the meat mixture in between your hands until a meatball is

formed. Place on a baking sheet lined with parchment paper.

4. Next to the meatballs, spread assorted veggies and lightly with drizzle oil, salt, and pepper.

5. Bake at for 15 minutes, or until meatballs are cooked through and vegetables are soft.

6. In a microwave-safe bowl, add all the ingredients for the orange sauce.

7. Stir orange sauce until well combined.

8. Microwave for 1 minute, stirring at 30 seconds.

9. Put veggies and meatballs over a bowl of rice and pour the sauce as desired.

10. Enjoy!

Meatless Paella

Ingredients

for 6 servings

- 2 tablespoons olive oil

- 1 medium yellow onion, minced

- 4 cloves garlic, minced

- 1 yellow bell pepper, cut into strips

- 1 red bell pepper, cut into strips

- 1 cup green beans (360 g), halved

- 1 ½ cups short grain white rice (300 g)

- ½ teaspoon smoked paprika

- ½ teaspoon sweet paprika

- 1 tablespoon tomato paste

- salt, to taste

- black pepper, to taste

- 14 oz diced tomato (395 g)

- 3 cups vegetable broth (720 mL)

- ½ teaspoon saffron thread, crumbled, or 1/2 tablespoon ground turmeric

- 2 bay leaves

- ½ cup frozen peas (75 g)

- ½ cup canned artichoke heart (85 g)

- ½ cup vegan chorizon (75 g), optional

- ½ cup fresh flat-leaf parsley (15 g), chopped

- 1 lemon, quartered, for garnish

Preparation

1. Heat the olive oil in a large skillet over medium heat.

2. Add the onion and cook until translucent, 3-4 minutes.

3. Add the garlic and cook for about 2 minutes until it is fragrant.

4. Add the yellow bell peppers, red bell peppers, and green beans. Cook stirring occasionally, for 5 minutes until tender.

5. Add the rice, smoked paprika, sweet paprika, tomato paste, salt, and pepper. Stir until incorporated. Cook for 1-2 minutes until the rice starts to sizzle.

6. Add the canned tomatoes. Cook for 5 minutes until the liquid has evaporated slightly.

7. Add the vegetable broth, saffron threads (crush the saffron threads between your fingertips), and bay leaves. Bring to a boil on high heat. Continue cooking, stirring occasionally, until most of the liquid is absorbed by the rice, about 10 minutes.

8. Add in the peas, artichokes, and sausage, if using. Cover the pan, reduce the heat to low, and cook for 10 minutes.

9. Remove the pan from the heat and let sit covered for 10 minutes.

10. Sprinkle the fresh parsley.

11. Enjoy!

Smoky Spiced Carrot Rice

Ingredients

for 2 servings

- 1 bunch carrot, peeled and sliced

- 1 tablespoon cooking oil, of preference, or water

- ½ white onion, diced

- ½ teaspoon salt

- ½ teaspoon pepper

- ½ teaspoon garlic powder

- 1 teaspoon smoked paprika

• fresh parsley, for garnish

Preparation

1. In a food processor, pulse the carrots until they reach your desired "rice" consistency.

2. In a large skillet over medium heat, heat oil, then add onions and let cook until translucent.

3. Add carrot rice, salt, pepper, garlic powder and paprika, and cook until the tender, stirring occasionally.

4. Garnish with parsley.

5. Enjoy!

Rainbow Veggie Roll

Ingredients

for 4 servings

- 2 cups sushi rice (460 g), cooked

- ¼ cup seasoned rice vinegar (60 mL)

- 4 half sheets sushi grade nori

- 1 avocado, thinly sliced

- 1 small cucumber, cut into matchsticks

- 1 cup bell pepper (100 g), assorted colors, cut into matchsticks

- sesame seed, optional

Preparation

1. Season the sushi rice with the rice vinegar, fanning and stirring until room temperature.

2. On the rolling mat place one sheet of nori with the rough side facing upwards.

3. Wet your hands and grab a handful of rice and place it on your nori. Sprinkle with seasame seeds (optional). Spread the rice evenly throughout the nori without smushing the rice down. Flip so the nori is facing upwards.

4. Arrange, in a horizontal row 1 inch (2.5 cm) from the bottom, bell peppers, cucumbers, and avocado slices.

5. Grabbing both nori and the mat, roll the mat over the filling so the extra space at the bottom touches the other side, squeezing down to make a nice tight roll. Squeeze down along the way to keep the roll from holding its shape.

6. Transfer the roll onto a cutting board. Rub a knife on a damp paper towel before slicing the roll into six equal portions.

7. Enjoy!

Sweet Sesame Dumplings (Tangyuan)

Ingredients

for 4 servings

Filling

- 1 cup black sesame seeds (150 g), toasted, ground

- ¼ cup powdered sugar (25 g)

- 1 ½ tablespoons unsalted butter

Dough

- 2 cups glutinous rice flour (250 g), plus more for dusting

- 1 cup warm water (240 mL)

For Cooking

- 2 tablespoons sugar

- 1 tablespoon osmanthus, dried flower

Preparation

1. Make the filling: In a medium bowl, combine the ground black sesame seeds, powdered sugar and melted butter. Mix until well combined. Roll 1 tablespoon scoops of the mixture into balls. Set aside.

2. Make the dough: Add the rice flour to a medium bowl. Gradually add the water and mix with your hands until the dough comes together.

3. On a lightly floured surface, turn out the dough. Shape into a ball and cut in half. Roll the dough into 2 logs, then cut into about 16 2-3-ounce (55G -85G) portions.

4. Flatten a dough portion in your palm and add a sesame ball to the center. Encase the filling with the dough and roll into a ball. Repeat with the remaining ingredients.

5. Bring a large pot of water to boil. Add the sugar and osmanthus flower. Drop the dumplings into the boiling water. Gently stir so they don't stick to the bottom of the pot. Cook until the dumplings float to the surface, then remove from the pot.

6. Serve the dumplings in a bowl with the cooking liquid.

7. Enjoy!

Gluten-Free Wild Rice Stuffing

Ingredients

for 10 servings

• 6 tablespoons unsalted butter, divided

• 1 lb Italian sausage (455 g), casings removed and broken up

• 1 medium white onion, diced

• 1 large carrot, diced

• 2 celery stalks, diced

• 1 ½ teaspoons kosher salt, divided

• 3 cloves garlic, mixed

• 1 tablespoon fresh thyme, leaves picked

• 5 leaves fresh sage, minced

- ½ teaspoon freshly ground black pepper

- 1 ¼ cups dried unsweetened cranberry (155 g)

- 1 cup pecan pieces (125 g), toasted

- ½ cup parmesan cheese (55 g)

- 4 cups wild rice medley (920 g), cooked

- 1 ¼ cups chicken stock (300 mL)

- 2 large eggs

- 1 large egg yolk

Preparation

1. Preheat the oven to 375°F (190°C). Grease a 9 x 13-inch (22.5 x 32.5 cm) baking dish with 1 tablespoon of butter.

2. In a medium pot over medium-high heat, cook the sausage until browned and cooked through,

about 8 minutes. Using a slotted spoon, transfer the sausage to a bowl, leaving the rendered fat behind in the pan. Set aside.

3. Lower the heat to medium and melt the remaining 5 tablespoons of butter in the pan with the sausage fat. Once the butter begins to bubble, add the onion, carrot, celery, and ½ teaspoon of salt. Cook for 5–8 minutes, until the onion is translucent and the carrots begin to soften.

4. Add the garlic, thyme leaves, sage, and black pepper and cook for 2–3 minutes, until the garlic is fragrant. Mix in the dried cranberries, pecans, Parmesan, rice, and sausage and stir well to combine. Remove the pot from the heat.

5. Transfer the stuffing mixture to the prepared baking dish.

6. In a liquid measuring cup, use a fork to whisk together the chicken stock, eggs, egg yolk, and remaining teaspoon of salt.

7. Pour the stock mixture evenly over the stuffing and stir to incorporate. Cover the dish with foil.

8. Bake the stuffing for 40 minutes. Remove the foil and bake for another 10 minutes, until slightly crispy on top. Remove the stuffing from the oven and let cool for 15–20 minutes before serving.

9. Serve warm.

10. Enjoy!

Gochujang Fried Fall Squash

Ingredients

for 8 servings

- 2 lb kobacha and delicata squash (910 g)

- 1 teaspoon kosher salt

- ½ teaspoon ground white pepper

- 1 teaspoon sesame oil

- 1 tablespoon grated fresh ginger

- ⅓ cup potato starch (40 g), plus more as needed

- ⅓ cup panko breadcrumbs (20 g)

- canola oil, for frying

Sauce

- 3 tablespoons unsalted butter

- 2 tablespoons minced garlic

- ¼ cup gochujang (25 g)

- 2 tablespoons ketchup

- ¼ cup honey (250 g)

- 2 tablespoons brown sugar

- 4 teaspoons rice vinegar

- 1 tablespoon soy sauce

- ½ teaspoon sesame oil

For Garnish

- sliced scallion, thinly

- sesame seed

Preparation

1. Prep the squash: Cut the kabocha squash in half through the stem and scoop out the seeds. Cut each half in half, then cut into ½-inch-thick slices. Transfer to a large bowl.

2. Cut the ends off the delicata squash, then slice in half lengthwise. Scoop out the seeds, then cut into ½-inch-thick slices. Add to the bowl with the kabocha squash. Season with the salt, white pepper, sesame oil, and ginger and toss to coat.

3. Make the sauce: Melt the butter in a small pot over medium heat. Add the garlic and let sizzle for a minute, until fragrant. Add the gochujang, ketchup, honey, brown sugar, rice vinegar, soy sauce, and sesame oil and whisk to combine. Bring to a simmer and cook for 2–3 minutes, then remove the pot from the heat.

4. In a medium bowl, stir together the potato starch and the panko. Sprinkle over the squash and toss to coat evenly (if the squash pieces do not have an even light white coating, add more potato starch and toss again). Press the panko onto the squash to adhere.

5. Heat a few inches of canola oil in a wok over medium-high heat until the temperature reaches 350°F (180°C). Place a wire rack over a sheet tray.

6. Working in batches to avoid overcrowding the pan, use tongs to carefully lower the squash pieces into the hot oil. Fry for 4–6 minutes, until dark golden brown. Transfer to the wire rack.

7. While the squash is still hot, toss in a large bowl with the sauce until well coated.

8. Garnished with sliced scallions and sesame seeds, then serve.

9. Enjoy!

Basil Lemongrass Curry

Ingredients

for 4 servings

• 4 stalks lemongrass

• ½ cup fresh basil (120 g)

• 2 ½ shallots, divided

• 1 ginger, roughly chopped - 1 inches (2.54 cm)

• 3 cloves garlic

• 2 teaspoons brown sugar

• ½ teaspoon turmeric

• ½ teaspoon ground coriander

• ½ teaspoon cumin

• ½ teaspoon salt

- ¼ teaspoon pepper

- 1 teaspoon red pepper flakes

- 2 cans reduced-fat coconut milk

- 1 tablespoon coconut oil

- 4 cups cooked rice (800 g)

- 1 lb shrimp (455 g), optional, shrimp, chicken

Any Vegetable toppings:

- bell pepper

- green onion

- broccoli

Preparation

1. Add chopped lemongrass, basil, 1 shallot, garlic, ginger, ground coriander, cumin, turmeric, salt, pepper, red pepper flakes, and brown sugar to a

food processor. Blend until a paste forms. (If difficult to combine, add 1 tbsp water to the mix and blend again).

2. Dice the remaining shallots and set aside.

3. Over medium heat, melt coconut oil in a large pan (big enough to hold 2 cans of coconut milk). Once the oil is hot and melted, add the basil lemongrass curry paste in. Let the curry paste bloom for 1 minute. Then add in the remaining chopped shallots and sauté until softened (2 minutes, approximately).

4. Pour in both cans of coconut milk and stir until combined. Cover and let curry reduce over medium heat for 20 minutes. Stir every so often. Season with salt and pepper.

5. While the curry simmers, prepare the meat and vegetables you will be using as desired.

6. Once the coconut curry has reduced and become thicker, begin assembling your dish. Pour the curry over a bed of rice, and top with any proteins and vegetables.

7. Serve and enjoy!

Baby Bok Choy Kimchi

Ingredients

for 4 servings

• 3 baby bok choys, (approximately 1.25 lbs)

• 2 teaspoons salt, separated and 1 teaspoon (Seperated)

• ⅓ cup rice (65 g), cooked

- ⅓ cup water (65 mL)

- 2 scallions, chopped in 2-inch (5 cm) lengths

- 2 tablespoons garlic

- 3 tablespoons gochugaru

- 3 teaspoons fish sauce

- 2 ½ tablespoons sugar (500 g)

Preparation

1. Rinse and cut the baby bok choy into fourths. Place bok choy in a large mixing bowl and sprinkle 2 tsp salt. Toss to evenly coat. Wait 30 minutes, then rinse and drain the bok choy. Return to the mixing bowl.

2. In a small blender, blend together the rice and water until it forms a smooth paste. Pour over the bok choy and mix together.

3. Add the rest of the ingredients and continue mixing gently, making sure all the ingredients get mixed thoroughly.

4. Store in an airtight container and let sit in the fridge for 1-2 hours to help flavors meld together. Eat.

5. Enjoy!

Fried Rice

Ingredients

for 10 servings

• 5 cups rice (1000 g)

• 1 tablespoon vegetable oil

- 1 ginger, peeled

- 3 cloves garlic, minced

- ½ red onion, diced

- mixed vegetable, frozen or fresh

- prefered seasoning

- butter

- 1 teaspoon lemon juice

- 1 tablespoon soy sauce, divided

- 1 teaspoon white pepper

- 1 teaspoon curry

- ½ teaspoon chicken bouillon powder

Preparation

1. Boil the rice in stock/broth and season ass desired.

2. Sauté ginger, 2 cloves of garlic, and red onion in vegetable oil on medium until fragrant. To this, add the mixed vegetables and seasonings of choice.

3. While vegetables are cooking, make a garlic butter paste with the remaining garlic and butter. To the paste, add lemon juice and ½ tbsp soy sauce and mix. Add 1 tbsp paste to the vegetables. Stir well on medium heat.

4. When veggies are done, remove from the pan and put in a separate bowl.

5. Put more oil in the pan and add the rice to the pan. Season rice with white pepper, curry, and chicken bouillon powder.

6. Add the garlic paste to rice and stir. Then, add vegetables, remaining soy sauce, and remaining garlic butter paste and stir well.

7. Serve warm.

Smoky Spiced Carrot Rice

Ingredients

for 2 servings

• 1 bunch carrot, peeled and sliced

• 1 tablespoon cooking oil, of preference, or water

• ½ white onion, diced

• ½ teaspoon salt

• ½ teaspoon pepper

• ½ teaspoon garlic powder

• 1 teaspoon smoked paprika

• fresh parsley, for garnish

Preparation

1. In a food processor, pulse the carrots until they reach your desired "rice" consistency.

2. In a large skillet over medium heat, heat oil, then add onions and let cook until translucent.

3. Add carrot rice, salt, pepper, garlic powder and paprika, and cook until the tender, stirring occasionally.

4. Garnish with parsley.

5. Enjoy!

Rainbow Veggie Roll

Ingredients

for 4 servings

• 2 cups sushi rice (460 g), cooked

• ¼ cup seasoned rice vinegar (60 mL)

• 4 half sheets sushi grade nori

• 1 avocado, thinly sliced

• 1 small cucumber, cut into matchsticks

• 1 cup bell pepper (100 g), assorted colors, cut into matchsticks

• sesame seed, optional

Preparation

1. Season the sushi rice with the rice vinegar, fanning and stirring until room temperature.

2. On the rolling mat place one sheet of nori with the rough side facing upwards.

3. Wet your hands and grab a handful of rice and place it on your nori. Sprinkle with seasame seeds (optional). Spread the rice evenly throughout the nori without smushing the rice down. Flip so the nori is facing upwards.

4. Arrange, in a horizontal row 1 inch (2.5 cm) from the bottom, bell peppers, cucumbers, and avocado slices.

5. Grabbing both nori and the mat, roll the mat over the filling so the extra space at the bottom touches the other side, squeezing down to make a nice tight roll. Squeeze down along the way to keep the roll from holding its shape.

6. Transfer the roll onto a cutting board. Rub a knife on a damp paper towel before slicing the roll into six equal portions.

7. Enjoy!

Sweet Sesame Dumplings (Tangyuan)

Ingredients

for 4 servings

Filling

- 1 cup black sesame seeds (150 g), toasted, ground

- ¼ cup powdered sugar (25 g)

- 1 ½ tablespoons unsalted butter

Dough

- 2 cups glutinous rice flour (250 g), plus more for dusting

- 1 cup warm water (240 mL)

For Cooking

• 2 tablespoons sugar

• 1 tablespoon osmanthus, dried flower

Preparation

1. Make the filling: In a medium bowl, combine the ground black sesame seeds, powdered sugar and melted butter. Mix until well combined. Roll 1 tablespoon scoops of the mixture into balls. Set aside.

2. Make the dough: Add the rice flour to a medium bowl. Gradually add the water and mix with your hands until the dough comes together.

3. On a lightly floured surface, turn out the dough. Shape into a ball and cut in half. Roll the dough into 2 logs, then cut into about 16 2-3-ounce (55G -85G) portions.

4. Flatten a dough portion in your palm and add a sesame ball to the center. Encase the filling with the dough and roll into a ball. Repeat with the remaining ingredients.

5. Bring a large pot of water to boil. Add the sugar and osmanthus flower. Drop the dumplings into the boiling water. Gently stir so they don't stick to the bottom of the pot. Cook until the dumplings float to the surface, then remove from the pot.

6. Serve the dumplings in a bowl with the cooking liquid.

7. Enjoy!

California Roll

Ingredients

for 4 servings

- 2 cups sushi rice (460 g), cooked

- ¼ cup seasoned rice vinegar (60 mL)

- 4 half sheets sushi grade nori

- 1 teaspoon sesame seed, optional

- 8 pieces imitation crab

- 1 small cucumber, cut into matchsticks

- 1 avocado, thinly sliced

Preparation

1. Season the sushi rice with the rice vinegar, fanning and stirring until room temperature.

2. On a rolling mat, place one sheet of nori with the rough side facing upwards.

3. Wet your hands and grab a handful of rice and place it on the nori. Spread the rice evenly throughout the nori without mashing the rice down. Season rice with a pinch of sesame seeds, if using, then flip it over so the nori is facing upwards.

4. Arrange, in a horizontal row 1 inch (2.5 cm) from the bottom, the crab followed by a row of avocado and a row of cucumber.

5. Grabbing both nori and the mat, roll the mat over the filling so the extra space at the bottom touches the other side, squeezing down to make a nice tight roll. Squeeze down along the way to keep the roll from holding its shape.

6. Transfer the roll onto a cutting board. Rub a knife on a damp paper towel before slicing the roll into six equal portions.

7. Enjoy!

Shrimp Tempura Rice Burger

Ingredients

for 3 servings

Tempura

• 1 egg

• 1 cup flour (120 g)

• ½ cup cold water (100 mL)

• flour, to cook

• 6 shrimps

• oil, to cook

Mayonnaise Sauce

• 3 tablespoons mayonnaise

• 1 tablespoon ketchup

• ½ tablespoon honey

• 1 teaspoon white vinegar

• 1 ¼ cups rice (300 g), cooked

• 2 tablespoons sesame oil, to cook

• green leaf lettuce, to taste

Preparation

1. Whisk the egg in a small bowl. Add 120 grams (1 cup) of flour and water. Whisk to combine. Cover with plastic wrap and transfer to the refrigerator.

2. Add flour to a shallow dish. Dip each shrimp in the flour, shaking off any excess.

3. Dip the floured shrimp into the batter.

4. Heat oil in a pot to 350°F (180°C).

5. Fry the shrimp until they float to the top and become golden brown in color. Use a slotted spoon to transfer the shrimp to a paper towel-lined plate to drain.

6. For the mayonnaise sauce, combine mayonnaise, ketchup, honey, and vinegar.

7. Line a ramekin with plastic wrap, and mold ¼ of the rice into a patty. Repeat until you have 6 rice "buns."

8. Heat a pan over medium-high heat and add a splash of sesame oil. Add the rice "buns" and cook until the outside is crispy, about 5 minutes.

9. Top the rice "bun" with a piece of green leaf lettuce, fried shrimps, mayonnaise sauce, and top with another rice "bun." Repeat with remaining ingredients.

10. Enjoy!

Fresh Fruit Sushi

Ingredients

for 20 pieces

• 1 ½ cups short grain rice (300 g)

- 2 cups water (480 mL)

- 3 tablespoons sugar

- ¼ teaspoon salt

- 1 cup coconut milk (240 mL)

- 1 ½ teaspoons vanilla

A variety of fruit

- pineapple

- strawberry

- mango

- kiwi

- 1 pt blackberry (475 g)

- raspberry

Preparation

1. In a medium pot combine the rice, water, sugar and salt. Cook on low heat for about 20 minutes or until all the rice absorbs the water.

2. Add the coconut milk and vanilla. The mixture should be moldable. Cook a few minutes longer if it's too runny.

3. Slice fruit of choice into long pieces.

4. *Note: Use a potato peeler to shave thin slices off the mango.

5. Lay a bamboo rolling pad on a counter top, and place a square of wax paper over top. Spread the rice about ½ inch (1 cm) thick over the paper into approximately a 7x5 inch (17x12 cm) rectangle.

6. Toast a ¼ cup (25g) of coconut shreds for 3 minutes.

7. Lay the fruit pieces on the rice, and roll up carefully. If rice sticks to the paper too much, try spreading it a little thicker.

8. Coat the rolls with either the mango slices, or the toasted coconut.

9. Slice each roll into 6 pieces.

10. With the rest of the rice, roll into balls (like nigiri).

11. Place thin slices of kiki or strawberries over top with half a blackberry on top to look like fish eggs.

12. Blend ¼ cup (25 g) raspberries with ¼ cup (60 ml) water to make a dipping sauce.

13. Enjoy!

Scallion Pizza Dough Pancake

Ingredients

for 4 pancakes

Scallion pancake

- pizza dough

- scallion

- sesame oil

- salt, to taste

- white pepper, to taste

Dipping sauce

- ⅓ cup soy sauce (80 mL)

- 2 tablespoons rice vinegar

- 1 teaspoon sriracha sauce

• 1 tablespoon garlic

• 1 tablespoon ginger

• 1 tablespoon sugar

• scallion, chopped

Preparation

1. Brush pizza dough with sesame oil. Liberally spread scallions. Salt and white pepper the pizza dough.

2. Cut pizza dough into 6 x 10 inch (15 x 25 cm) pieces. Roll and coil. Rest covered with a damp towel for an hour.

3. After an hour, flatten each coil of dough, roll out as flat as possible. Fry on medium heat until both sides are golden brown (5 minutes). Then cut into quarters.

4. Mix the **Ingredients** for the dipping sauce into a small bowl. Serve.

5. Enjoy!

Chewy Oatmeal Breakfast Bars To-go

Ingredients

for 8 servings

• 1 cup almond butter (240 g)

• ½ cup maple syrup (110 g)

• ½ cup almond milk (120 mL)

• 1 teaspoon vanilla

• 2 ½ cups rolled oats (250 g)

- 1 cup brown rice cereal (30 g)

- ½ cup slivered almond (35 g)

- ½ cup dried cranberry (65 g)

- ½ cup dark chocolate (85 g)

Drizzle

- ¼ cup dark chocolate (40 g), melted

Preparation

1. Preheat oven to 325°F (160°C).

2. Combine wet **Ingredients** together in a large bowl.

3. Then add in all the remaining dry ingredients.

4. Add mixture into a 8x8 inch (20x20 cm) baking pan lined with greased parchment paper. Firmly press down mixture until it is one smooth layer. (If

you grease the spatula as well it will prevent the mixture from sticking to it!)

5. Bake 15-20 minutes, or until golden brown. Let cool 10 minutes.

6. Drizzle top with melted dark chocolate. Chill for 30 minutes, or until dark chocolate is solid.

7. Cut into 8 equal pieces.

8. Wrap each bar in parchment paper or foil.

9. Store in the freezer for up to 3 months or in the refrigerator up to 1 week.

10. Enjoy!

Blueberry Chocolate Energy Bars

Ingredients

for 16 bars

• 1 cup raw almond (140 g)

• 1 cup raw walnut (100 g)

• 2 ½ cups pitted date (425 g), roughly chopped

• 1 teaspoon salt, plus more to taste

• ½ cup water (120 mL)

• 1 ½ cups brown rice cereal (45 g)

• 1 ½ cups old fashion oat (150 g)

• ½ cup dried blueberry (50 g)

• ½ tablespoon cinnamon

• 3 cups dark chocolate (510 g), chopped

• 2 tablespoons coconut oil

Preparation

1. Preheat the oven to 350°F (180°C). Line a baking sheet with parchment paper.

2. Spread the almonds on one half of the baking sheet and the walnuts on the other half.

3. Toast for 10-15 minutes, or until lightly browned and fragrant. Let cool 20 minutes before roughly chopping.

4. In a food processor or blender, combine the dates, salt, and water, and process until well-combined.

5. Transfer the date mixture to a large bowl and add the brown rice cereal, oats, blueberries, cinnamon, and salt. Stir until well-combined. Add the chopped nuts and fold to combine.

6. Transfer the mixture to a parchment-lined baking sheet and spread flat with a spatula.

7. Cover with plastic wrap and chill in the fridge for 30-45 minutes to set.

8. In a large bowl, combine the chocolate and coconut oil, and microwave for 1½ minutes, stirring every 30 seconds, until melted and smooth

9. Pour ⅔ of the melted chocolate over the bars and spread evenly. Cover with plastic wrap and freeze for 10 minutes, or until the chocolate is set.

10. Invert the bars onto a cutting board and remove the parchment paper. Drizzle the remaining chocolate over the top. Return to the freezer for 10 minutes, until the chocolate is set.

11. Cut into 16 bars. Wrap individually in parchment paper and store in the fridge or freezer until ready to eat.

12. Enjoy!

Unicorn Cookies

Ingredients

for 30 cookies

• 16 tablespoons unsalted butter

• 1 cup granulated sugar (200 g)

• ⅔ cup light brown sugar (150 g), packed

• 1 tablespoon corn syrup

• 2 large eggs

• ½ teaspoon vanilla extract

• 2 cups all purpose flour (250 g)

• ½ teaspoon baking powder

• ¼ teaspoon baking soda

• 1 teaspoon kosher salt

• ¾ cup white chocolate chip (130 g)

• ½ cup rainbow sprinkles (80 g)

• ⅓ cup rolled oats (25 g)

• 1 cup sweetened rice cereal (30 g)

• 1 cup fruit shaped cereal (30 g)

• 30 cone shaped corn chips, for garnish

Preparation

1. In a large bowl with an electric hand mixer or in a stand mixer fitted with the paddle attachment, cream together the butter, granulated sugar, brown

sugar, and corn syrup until light and fluffy, about 5 minutes.

2. Scrape down the sides of the bowl with a rubber spatula, then add the eggs and vanilla. Beat for 3 minutes, or until fully incorporated.

3. Add the flour, baking powder, baking soda, and salt and mix just until the dough comes together. Do not overmix.

4. Scrape down the sides of the bowl again, then fold in the white chocolate chips, sprinkles, oats, rice cereal, and fruit-shaped cereal.

5. Using an ice cream scoop or ¼ measuring cup (60 grams), scoop the dough onto a parchment-lined baking sheet. Cover with plastic wrap and refrigerate for at least 1 hour, or up to a 1 week.

6. Preheat the oven to 350°F (180°C). Line baking sheets with parchment paper.

7. Arrange the chilled dough balls 4 inches (10 cm) apart on the prepared baking sheets.

8. Bake for 6 minutes, then remove the cookies from the oven and place a corn chip in the center of each cookie to resemble a unicorn horn. Return to the oven for 6-8 minutes more, until lightly browned around the edges.

9. Let the cookies cool completely on the baking sheets before serving. The cookies will keep in an airtight container at room temperature for 5 days, or in the freezer for up to 1 month.

10. Enjoy!

Jasmine's Snack Board

Ingredients

for 4 servings

Prawn Crackers

• 2 cups canola oil (480 mL), for frying

• 1 box prawn-flavored chips

Spam Musubi

• 2 tablespoons canola oil

• ½ can Spam®, halved lengthwise

• 2 tablespoons water

• 2 tablespoons soy sauce

• 2 tablespoons sugar, plus 2 teaspoons, divided

• ½ teaspoon kosher salt

• 2 tablespoons rice vinegar

• 1 ⅓ cups sushi rice (265 g), cooked

• 4 strips nori, 2 in (5 cm)

California Roll

• canola oil, for greasing

• 2 cups sushi rice (400 g), cooked, seasoned with 2 tablespoons of rice vinegar

• 8 pieces imitation crab

• 1 avocado, thinly sliced

• 1 small cucumber, cut into machsticks

• 4 sheets sushi-grade nori, 8½ x 7½

Assembly

• 1 package pan-fried dumplings, 24 ounce (700 G)

• 2 cups garlic edamame (320 g)

- 4 scallion pancakes, cut into triangles

- 1 large red dragon fruit, peeled and diced

- 4 pineapple cakes

- 4 probiotic yogurt drinks

- 8 pieces assorted mochi

- 1 loaf mujigae-tteok loaf, sliced

- 2 strawberry flavored Hello Panda cookies, 9 ounce (260 grams)

- 4 choco pies

- 1 cara cara orange, large, sliced

- 2 Mandarin orange slices

- 1 large asian pear, sliced

Preparation

1. Make the prawn crackers: Heat the oil in a large heavy-bottomed pan over medium heat until the temperature reaches 325°F (160°C). Line a plate with paper towels and set nearby.

2. Place 8–10 chips in a slotted spoon or spider. Gently lower them into the hot oil and stir gently. As the chips begin to float to the surface, quickly remove from the oil before they scorch or burn. Carefully shake off any excess oil, and then place on the lined plate. Continue frying the remaining chips.

3. Make the spam musubi: Heat the canola oil in a large nonstick skillet over medium-high heat. Add the Spam and cook for 2–3 minutes per side, until golden brown and crispy.

4. In a small bowl, whisk together the water, soy sauce, and 2 tablespoons of sugar.

5. Reduce the heat to low and pour the soy sauce mixture into the skillet. Cook until the sauce is bubbly and thick and coats the Spam evenly, turning as needed, about 5 minutes total. Remove the pan from the heat.

6. In a medium bowl, whisk together the remaining 2 teaspoons sugar, salt, and vinegar. Add the cooked sushi rice and stir to combine.

7. Lay a strip of nori, shiny side down, on a clean surface. Place the box of the musubi press on top. Add ⅓ cup of the seasoned rice to the box and press down with the plunger. Lay a piece of Spam on top of the rice and press down firmly. Lift the box to release the Spam and rice. Wrap the nori around the stack, using a wet finger to seal the nori.

8. Make the California rolls: Lightly grease the inner chamber of a sushi bazooka with canola oil.

9. Add ½ cup of the seasoned sushi rice to each half of the inner chamber and use the plunger to create a divot down the length of each side of rice. Arrange half of the crab, avocado, and cucumber in a horizontal row on one side of the rice. Carefully close the bazooka.

10. Lay a piece of nori, shiny side down, on the sushi mat. Turn the plunger 5 times, then firmly press to release the roll onto one end of the nori. Tightly roll the nori around the rice to completely encase the roll. Transfer the roll to a cutting board. Rub a knife on a damp paper towel before slicing the roll crosswise into 6 equal pieces. Repeat with the remaining ingredients to make another roll.

11. Assemble the board: Place the prawn crackers, musubi, and California rolls in the center of a turntable. Arrange the pan-fried dumplings, garlic edamame, scallion pancakes, dragonfruit,

pineapple cakes, probiotic yogurt drinks, mochi, mujigae-tteok, Hello Panda cookies, Choco pies, Cara Cara and Mandarin oranges, and Asian pears around the edges.

12. Enjoy!

Nobu-Style Cup Sushi

Ingredients

for 10 servings

Rice

• 5 cups sushi rice (1 kg)

• 5 cups water (1 L)

Sushi Vinegar

- 1 ¼ cups red vinegar (300 mL), Akazu, divided to 250ml and 50 ml

- ½ cup monkfruit sweetener (160 g)

- ¼ cup salt (60 g)

- ¼ cup mirin (20 mL)

- 2-inch square piece of kombu

Toppings

- soy sauce

- sliced sushi-grade tuna

- sliced sushi-grade yellowtail

- sliced sushi-grade red snapper

- sliced sushi-grade salmon

- sliced sushi-grade scallop

- sushi-grade salmon roe

- ½ cup cooked crab (225 g)

- sushi-grade sea urchin

- sushi-grade squid

- ½ cup cooked shrimp (165 g)

- crumbled nori

- chopped fresh cilantro

- sliced jalapeño

- caviar

- masago

Preparation

1. Place the rice in a sieve and rinse under water 4-5 times, until the water is clear.

2. Place the rice and water in a pot and bring to a boil. Once the water is at a rolling boil, put a lid on

top and cook for 15 minutes on low heat. Turn off the heat and let it sit for 10 minutes.

3. In a small saucepan over medium heat, add 250ml (1 cup) red vinegar, monk fruit sweetener, salt, and mirin and Kombu. Once the sweetner and salt are dissolved add 50ml (¼ cup) of the vinegar. Set aside to cool to room temperature.

4. Place the cooked rice in a wooden tub or a large bowl. Sprinkle 150ml (½ cup) sushi vinegar evenly over the rice while the rice is still hot and mix with a wooden spoon. Cover the rice with a wet tea towel and cool until close to body temperature. Save leftover sushi vinegar for next time.

5. Place 1-2 tablespoons of rice in a small cup. Spray soy sauce on the rice. Sprinkle some crumbled seaweed on top. Top with thinly sliced fresh seafood or your favorite toppings.

6. Enjoy!

Glutinous Rice Balls (Tang Yuan)

Ingredients

for 20 balls

Fillings

• ¼ cup black sesame seeds (35 g)

• ¼ cup unsalted peanuts (30 g)

• 4 tablespoons granulated sugar, divided

• 2 tablespoons unsalted butter, room temperature

Brown Sugar Ginger Syrup

• 2 cups water (480 mL)

• ½ cup brown sugar (100 g)

• 2 tablespoons fresh ginger, peeled and sliced

Dough

• 1 ¼ cups glutinous rice flour (155 g), ¼ cup boiling water (60 ml) ¼ cup room temperature water (60 ml)

• pink food coloring

Preparation

1. Make the fillings: Add the sesame seeds to a small nonstick pan. Cook over low heat, stirring often, until they start to smell nutty, 3–4 minutes.

2. Transfer the sesame seeds to a small food processor with 2 tablespoons of sugar. Process until the seeds break down into a thick, cohesive paste. Add 1 tablespoon of butter and process until smooth. Transfer to an airtight container and

refrigerate until hardened, at least 1 hour or up to 4 days.

3. Clean the bowl of the food processor, then repeat the toasting and blending process with the peanuts, remaining 2 tablespoons of sugar, and remaining tablespoon of butter. Transfer to an airtight container and refrigerate until hardened, at least 1 hour or up to 4 days.

4. Divide the sesame paste into 10 equal portions, about 1½ teaspoons each. Repeat with the peanut paste. Freeze until ready to use.

5. Make the brown sugar ginger syrup: Add the water, brown sugar, and ginger to a small saucepan. Cook over medium-low heat, stirring occasionally, until the sugar is dissolved, 3–5 minutes. Remove the pan from the heat and let cool to room temperature, then refrigerate until ready to serve.

(Alternatively, if you prefer to serve the tang yuan in hot syrup, cover to keep warm until ready to serve.)

6. Make the dough: Add the glutinous rice flour to a large bowl. Slowly pour in the boiling water and whisk until combined. Slowly pour in the room temperature water and stir with a rubber spatula until the dough comes together. Turn the dough out onto a clean surface and knead with your hands until smooth and soft, 2–3 minutes.

7. Divide the dough in 2 portions. Set one portion aside and cover with a damp paper towel, then return the other portion to the bowl used to make the dough. Add a couple of drops of pink food coloring and knead with your hands (wear latex gloves to avoid dyeing your hands pink) until the color is evenly distributed.

8. Roll each color of dough into 10 equal balls, about 1 tablespoon each. Place on a tray and cover with a damp paper towel to keep from drying out as you roll.

9. Working one at a time, flatten each dough ball into a 2-inch circle. Press your thumb into the center to make a divot, then add one of the chilled filling balls to the divot and pull the dough around to encase. Roll a few times to create a smooth, uniform round. Repeat with the remaining dough and fillings, covering the filled tang yuan with a damp paper towel as you finish.

10. Bring a large pot of water to a boil. If serving cold, prepare an ice bath in a medium bowl and set nearby. Add about 6 tang yuan and immediately stir to prevent sticking. Cook until they start to float, about 3 minutes, then cook for 1 minute more. Use a slotted spoon to remove from the water and

transfer to the ice bath, if applicable. Transfer to a serving bowl. Repeat with the remaining tang yuan.

11. Pour the chilled brown sugar ginger syrup over the tang yuan and serve immediately.

12. Enjoy!

Chocolate Horchata Popsicles Planet Oat

Ingredients

for 12 servings

• 1 small mexican cinnamon stick

• ½ cup white rice (120 mL)

• 5 cups Planet Oat® Dark Chocolate Oatmilk (1 L)

- ¼ cup sugar (25 g)

- 1 teaspoon vanilla extract

- 1 ½ tablespoons ground cinnamon

- ¾ cup dark chocolate (150 g), chopped, 60%

Toppings (Optional)

- ½ cup toasted coconut flakes (50 g), plus 2 tablespoons

- ½ cup toasted sliced almonds (60 g), plus 2 tablespoons

Equipment

- 12 ice pop sticks

- 2 ice pop molds, 6 count

Preparation

1. In a medium pot over medium-low heat, toast the cinnamon stick(s) for 1 minute, or until fragrant. Add the white rice and toast for another minute.

2. Add the Planet Oat® Dark Chocolate Oatmilk, sugar, vanilla, and ground cinnamon. Simmer for about 3 minutes, or until the cinnamon is fragrant, stirring occasionally. Remove the pot from the heat and let the chocolate horchata chill in the refrigerator for 8 hours or overnight. Discard the Mexican cinnamon stick and blend the horchata on high speed for 30–60 seconds, or until finely pulverized.

3. Strain the liquid into a fine mesh strainer over a large measuring cup. Divide the chocolate horchata evenly between 2 6-count ice pop molds. Freeze for 30–45 minutes, until slightly solidified. Insert the sticks into the center of the pops, then return to the freezer for 8 hours, or overnight.

4. Add the dark chocolate to a microwave-safe bowl and microwave for 30–60 seconds, until melted. Let cool slightly.

5. If using, add the toasted coconut flakes and sliced almonds to 2 separate shallow bowls.

6. Remove the ice pops from the freezer and remove from the molds. Dip the top third of each pop in the melted dark chocolate, then immediately dip in the coconut flakes or almonds. Lay the pops on a plate and freeze for 5 minutes before serving.

7. Enjoy!

Gochujang Fried Fall Squash

Ingredients

for 8 servings

• 2 lb kobacha and delicata squash (910 g)

• 1 teaspoon kosher salt

• ½ teaspoon ground white pepper

• 1 teaspoon sesame oil

• 1 tablespoon grated fresh ginger

• ⅓ cup potato starch (40 g), plus more as needed

• ⅓ cup panko breadcrumbs (20 g)

• canola oil, for frying

Sauce

• 3 tablespoons unsalted butter

• 2 tablespoons minced garlic

• ¼ cup gochujang (25 g)

• 2 tablespoons ketchup

• ¼ cup honey (250 g)

• 2 tablespoons brown sugar

• 4 teaspoons rice vinegar

• 1 tablespoon soy sauce

• ½ teaspoon sesame oil

For Garnish

• sliced scallion, thinly

• sesame seed

Preparation

1. Prep the squash: Cut the kabocha squash in half through the stem and scoop out the seeds. Cut each half in half, then cut into ½-inch-thick slices. Transfer to a large bowl.

2. Cut the ends off the delicata squash, then slice in half lengthwise. Scoop out the seeds, then cut into ½-inch-thick slices. Add to the bowl with the kabocha squash. Season with the salt, white pepper, sesame oil, and ginger and toss to coat.

3. Make the sauce: Melt the butter in a small pot over medium heat. Add the garlic and let sizzle for a minute, until fragrant. Add the gochujang, ketchup, honey, brown sugar, rice vinegar, soy sauce, and sesame oil and whisk to combine. Bring to a simmer and cook for 2–3 minutes, then remove the pot from the heat.

4. In a medium bowl, stir together the potato starch and the panko. Sprinkle over the squash and toss to coat evenly (if the squash pieces do not have an even light white coating, add more potato starch and toss again). Press the panko onto the squash to adhere.

5. Heat a few inches of canola oil in a wok over medium-high heat until the temperature reaches 350°F (180°C). Place a wire rack over a sheet tray.

6. Working in batches to avoid overcrowding the pan, use tongs to carefully lower the squash pieces into the hot oil. Fry for 4–6 minutes, until dark golden brown. Transfer to the wire rack.

7. While the squash is still hot, toss in a large bowl with the sauce until well coated.

8. Garnished with sliced scallions and sesame seeds, then serve.

9. Enjoy!

Baby Bok Choy Kimchi

Ingredients

for 4 servings

• 3 baby bok choys, (approximately 1.25 lbs)

• 2 teaspoons salt, separated and 1 teaspoon (Seperated)

• ⅓ cup rice (65 g), cooked

• ⅓ cup water (65 mL)

• 2 scallions, chopped in 2-inch (5 cm) lengths

• 2 tablespoons garlic

• 3 tablespoons gochugaru

• 3 teaspoons fish sauce

• 2 ½ tablespoons sugar (500 g)

Preparation

1. Rinse and cut the baby bok choy into fourths. Place bok choy in a large mixing bowl and sprinkle 2 tsp salt. Toss to evenly coat. Wait 30 minutes, then rinse and drain the bok choy. Return to the mixing bowl.

2. In a small blender, blend together the rice and water until it forms a smooth paste. Pour over the bok choy and mix together.

3. Add the rest of the ingredients and continue mixing gently, making sure all the ingredients get mixed thoroughly.

4. Store in an airtight container and let sit in the fridge for 1-2 hours to help flavors meld together. Eat.

5. Enjoy!

CHAPTER VI: A FINAL NOTE!

I know that you have a lot on your plate with job, family, and other responsibilities. It might be difficult to lose weight because of the time and effort it requires. But I want you to know that it is possible, and that I am here to provide you all the help and encouragement you require.

First and first, I want to stress the importance of remembering that your motivation to lose weight stems from a desire to improve your health and well-being, not just your appearance. Your dedication to your health is demonstrated by your willingness to explore taking this action.

Despite your busy schedule, here are some tips and words of encouragement to help you lose weight.:

- Recognizing that losing weight takes time, pace yourself by setting small, manageable objectives. Honor even the smallest of gains along the path.

- Include self-care as a mandatory element of your schedule. It might be anything as simple as a 20-minute stroll, a balanced dinner, or a few moments of meditation. Keep in mind that self-care is not an option, but a need.

- Fast food and pre-packaged meals are common choices for busy folks. Spend some time on the weekend preparing healthy meals for the week ahead. Time-poor people might benefit from planning ahead and preparing healthful meals that can be frozen for use throughout the week.

- Drink lots of water throughout the day to maintain your body's water balance. Our bodies can be fooled into munching when they think they're thirsty instead of hungry.

- Watch what you put into your body. Don't munch away at your desk or the TV screen. Take your time and enjoy your food. Knowing when you're full is an important step in controlling your weight.

- Getting to the gym may be difficult, but there are other options for maintaining physical fitness. Avoid using the elevator and opt for short walks or a quick at-home workout instead.

- Get a good night's rest. Getting too little sleep might make you gain weight. Develop some soothing habits for before bed to help you wind down and get to sleep more quickly.

- You might want to join a support group or find a friend to lose weight together. Motivation and responsibility may be gained via telling people about your experience.

- Keep in mind that everyone makes mistakes sometimes. The path to losing weight is not always straight. The way you deal with failure is the most important thing. Focus on self-compassion rather than self-criticism to help you get back on track.

- Talk to a dietitian or fitness expert if you can. They can help you choose a strategy that works for you and provide you expert guidance.

- Use a notebook or a weight loss app to record your daily diet and activity levels, as well as your progress toward your goal. Having your successes written down might be an inspiration boost.

- Last but not least, trust that you have what it takes to lose weight. If you ever find yourself questioning your decision to go on this adventure, just think back to your original motivation.

Despite your hectic schedule, I'm confident in your ability to complete this mission. When it comes to losing weight, it's not simply about stopping at the gym and hoping for the best. You have limitless potential, and I will be here to cheer you on as you explore it. I am here for you whenever you need someone to vent to, celebrate with, or lean on during the terrible times.